Effective Presentations for Health Care Professionals

For my family, who taught me that what matters is not what happens but how you handle it

Effective Presentations for Health Care Professionals

Lisa Hadfield-Law RGN

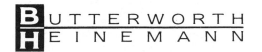

OXFORD AUCKLAND BOSTON JOHANNESBURG MELBOURNE NEW DELHI

Butterworth-Heinemann
Linacre House, Jordan Hill, Oxford OX2 8DP
225 Wildwood Avenue, Woburn, MA 01801-2041
A division of Reed Educational and Professional Publishing Ltd

R A member of the Reed Elsevier plc group

First Published 1999

British Library Cataloguing in Publication Data
A catalogue record for this book is available from the British Library.

Library of Congress Cataloguing in Publication Data
A catalogue record for this book is available from the Library of
Congress.

ISBN 0 7506 3843 5

Typeset by David Gregson Associates, Beccles, Suffolk
Printed in Great Britain by Biddles Ltd, Guildford and Kings Lynn

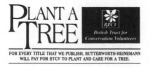

Contents

Preface

Effective Presentations for Health Care Professionals is the product of fifteen years of making presentations and training others to do so. It is a collection of the most up-to-date strategies and tips, which have been used by many, around the world, who have been generous with their ideas and feedback. I have drawn extensively on my own experiences and what has worked for me, for which I make no apology.

I would be grateful for any feedback from you, in the form of ideas, comments, criticisms or suggestions. This will help me to make improvements in the future.

The central themes of the book have their roots in my coaching of expert and novice presenters. This small volume cannot hope to cover all aspects of presenting, but it does address the issues which have been raised most often by participants in my seminars. Presenting is a practical skill and the most important part of acquiring the skill is practice.

So this book is only a start. The most important part of reading the book, is to close it at the end and to start putting the principles into practice.

1 Introduction

Good public speaking can be learned

Effective presentation involves the ability to communicate a message to an audience, which produces a desired change in understanding or opinion. It sounds easy enough for those working in the caring professions, who often pride themselves on excellent communication skills. However, for many, the prospect of standing up and speaking in front of others is terrifying. Speaking in public comes naturally to few, but involves skills which can be learned. Such skills are an important part of work in any clinical, research, managerial or educational position. Whether we like it or not, others often judge our competence based on our presentation skills.

It is so interesting to see the wonderful advances made in health care and the technology associated with it. It is surprising, though, that little has changed in the field of making presentations. Standards associated with this activity have become more of a challenge with the development of television. By pressing a button we can immediately tune in to slick presenters, delivering professional presentations. Your posture, body language, facial expression, use of voice and appearance all matter. These factors can work in your favour, with some planning, practise and feedback. I will raise issues to make the preparation and delivery of presentations easier, more certain and more fun, as well as making sure you get your message across to the audience.

You may be wondering what makes me such an expert. Like most successful coaches, the art of presenting does not come naturally to me. Throughout my career I have felt passionately about excellent patient care and the contribution of nursing. I have always been impressed by those

Any man who
never steps on
anyone else's
toes is standing
still.

Winston Churchill

willing to stand up in front of professional colleagues, to share what they are doing, and to make a contribution to raising standards of care.

Despite the commitment to speak about what I do, there have been times during my working life when I have been crippled by anxiety. On one occasion my mind went blank in front of a television audience of millions; on another I vomited behind a lectern on the stage; and to complete this catalogue of disasters, I fainted (not role playing) in front of yet another group of nurses and doctors, who were learning how to handle difficult situations during training sessions. However, I remind myself that making presentations involves skills which come naturally to few, but can be learned. I truly believe that what we have to share, as health care professionals, is too important to keep to ourselves, just because we are anxious about speaking in public. If we really are committed to putting patients first, we must be prepared to tell others about what we do.

This raises another issue. I am surprised by the occasional colleague who seems to take every opportunity, informally, to tell others about their ideas and how well they are doing, but does not use any formal channel to do so. They then express resentment when others take the time to make a presentation or write about what they do. It is pointless to grumble that you established case management on an orthopaedic ward long before Staff Nurse Rising Starr filled in his first fluid balance chart. If you want credit for success, you need to talk or write about it formally. For those of you who do take the risk, remember the words of Winston Churchill Any man who never steps on anyone else's toes is standing still.

Of course success breeds success. By promoting yourself, your specialty and your profession with words, either spoken or written, you will add to your curriculum vitae (CV). A good CV will help you put a foot onto the career ladder. However, a CV is only part of recruitment and selection. Many interviews for clinical positions, even at a comparatively junior level, now require a presentation as part of the process. It is said that more people have talked their way to the top of the ladder than any other way.

For those of you who make presentations regularly, how much feedback have you had? If you deliver a poor presentation lasting 30 minutes, to an audience of 200, you have wasted at least 30 minutes of your own time and over four days of theirs. Remember, no matter what field

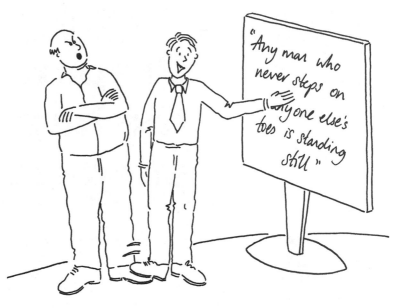

"Any man who never steps on anyone else's toes is standing still"

Put all you learn into practice

you work in, you need to be able to present your ideas effectively to others. You will only know how effective you are, by eliciting feedback directly from the audience or by reviewing your performance with a colleague or on video camera.

I have written this book to convince you of the importance of being able to put your ideas across to others, and to help you to inform, persuade or entertain, and will provide you with invaluable tips on how to do so. However, the most important part of reading this book is to put all you learn into practice afterwards. You do not play good tennis by reading about it. You do not have to start by entertaining hundreds with your sparkling wit after dinner, or at a formal international conference. Start with a small group of work colleagues, family or friends.

Remember that the audience will almost always want you to succeed. Few enjoy watching others struggle. Let us keep it in perspective:

When Moses presented the Ten Commandments to his people he said: 'O my Lord, I am not eloquent, neither heretofore, nor since thou hast spoken unto thy servant: but I am slow of speech and of a slow tongue'

Exodus 2

- Great presenters are not born, they make themselves.
- Spontaneity is the product of disciplined preparation.
- Compared to eternity it is small fry.

Do not be seduced into focusing on yourself and your performance, remember that your priority must be about the contribution your presentation can make.

2 Preparation is the key to success

There is no doubt that most of us who have had uncomfortable experiences when speaking, have not prepared properly. Winston Churchill claimed to prepare for an hour for every minute he spoke in public. It is not just the time spent preparing, but what you do during that time. Faced with the prospect of presenting, many will leave preparation to the last minute and will then rush to the library to find anything ever written about their chosen area. Such methods are doomed to failure. Few, if any, management skills come down to one magic formula, but with presentations, preparation comes close.

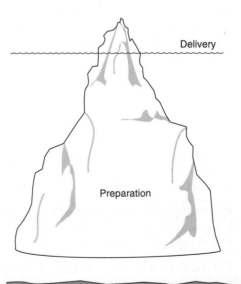

Figure 2.1 The stages involved in making a presentation resemble an iceberg – the largest proportion of effort lies below the surface.

Ask some questions first

Preparation should begin the minute you are asked, or you ask, to speak. I try to do a little work on each presentation, every day, until I give it. Answers to the following questions need to be written down straight away:

1 **Who are you speaking to?** What background do they have? Are they a small group of experienced physiotherapists or a hundred medical students. Untrained speakers sometimes create one 'talk' and deliver it the same way, no matter what type of audience they have. This failure to tailor the presentation to the listener will often fail.

2 **How many?** This will affect how you deliver your presentation, particularly when planning visual aids. It is also disconcerting to arrive at a venue with a carousel full of slides to be met by a group of three, or to prepare a flip chart for an audience of 200.

3 **What are the gender and age ranges?** If the majority of the audience are women in their twenties, then they will probably know who Leonardo DiCaprio is. However, they may not know who Audie Murphy was. Groups of men in their forties or fifties may be familiar with David Duckham and his achievements, but would not know who Boyzone are. This is worth considering when planning examples and illustrations. Audiences appreciate efforts to use meaningful illustrations.

4 **Do they have the choice of attending?** You may need to spend a little more time encouraging audiences to listen to what you have to say if they have been forced to attend.

5 **What will they want from you?** You need to ask the organizers what is required by them first of all. You can then start to imagine what the audience will expect. Occasionally I have contacted people who I know will be in the audience, to ask them what they would like to cover. This has proved very fruitful.

6 **What is the aim and the theme of the meeting?** Once you know the direction, you can begin to fit your section into it.

7 **Are there any current problems or concerns for the group?** If you are addressing a group of occupational therapists facing redundancy in the near future,

there may be sensitive issues to be aware of. You will face a frosty reception if you are speaking about multiskilling. However, forewarned is forearmed.

8 **Are there any issues to avoid, if so, why?** When lecturing to a group from one unit, I launched into a section of a medico-legal session concerned with taking out a grievance. I lost the audience very quickly to whispers and distraction as soon as I tried to move on. This particular team had taken out a grievance against the management of the Trust and, once I had shifted the focus from me onto their main concern, I found it almost impossible to retrieve the session. Had I known in advance, I could have avoided the issue and hence the distraction.

9 **Who is speaking before you and what about?** When you have sat at the front of an audience before your presentation to hear your content covered, almost verbatim and unwittingly, by a previous speaker, you will always take measures to prevent the situation occurring again. Having perused the programme, I make every effort to contact other speakers to ascertain what they plan to cover.

10 **How much time do you have?** Always make sure the organizers are specific. It is impossible to plan to 'Take as much time as you need'. 'Half an hour to an hour' is non-specific too.

11 **If I am introduced late, do I shorten the presentation or extend the schedule?** You may need to recheck this just before you speak, but quietly and without involving the audience.

12 **Where is the venue and how do I get there?** I once organized a conference at St Bartholomew's Hospital in London whilst I was working in Oxford. I had booked speakers a year beforehand and had written to them several times about visual aid requirements, catering, travel expenses, who would meet them and where. On the morning of the conference I was paged by one of the speakers who was in the centre of Oxford looking for St Bartholomew's Hospital. I was to blame, as I had written to him from an Oxford address and it did not occur to him that I would be arranging the conference elsewhere. The speaker never did make his presentation, which was a waste. He had worked hard on it, and the content was of great interest to the delegates.

13 Who is the contact and what is their telephone number? Thankfully the speaker in the wrong city had several contact numbers and was able to contact us easily. You need to know who to contact for any routine queries and in an emergency, should one arise.

Once you have the answers to all these questions, write them down. Do not try to commit them to memory, they are bound to get lost, and you will need them a month or even a year later.

Where do you start?

Conceive the conclusion

The conclusion is the last part of any presentation the audience will hear and the part they are most likely to remember. Many successful barristers exploit this. They write their final argument first, and then line up the evidence that best supports the facts they must prove to the jury. Accomplished speakers, such as Gladstone, wrote down and memorized the exact words of their closings.

Studies show that the audience forget around 50 per cent of what you tell them within 24 hours, and 90 per cent within two weeks. It may be helpful to ask yourself the following questions.

1 When I finish my presentation I want the audience to _____.

2 During the presentation I want to appear

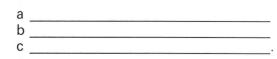

3 Two weeks later I want the audience to remember _____.

As soon as you have agreed to make a presentation, start a file. A simple document wallet will do. You can then place all the information you gather in one accessible place. However, it is still not yet time to rush to the library. Take a while first to think about your purpose. What do you want your audience to do, think, feel or know after your time slot is over? 'Begin with the end in mind' (Covey, 1989).

A speech is like a love affair. Any fool can start it, but to end it requires considerable skill

Lord Moncrief

Take a piece of paper and write in one sentence the major point of your presentation. Once you have decided what your 'end' will be, you can write your closing remarks. Although this may not be the approach you would usually take, you will find it much easier to stay focused and achieve your aim.

The conclusion should take about 5–10 per cent of the overall presentation time. You can use it as the opportunity to summarize, provide closure, make a good last impression and to motivate your audience. The three to five salient points should be repeated. Most people need to hear a point at least seven times before it is lodged in their mind.

It is important to signal that you are nearing the end of your talk. As soon as the audience hear 'In conclusion . . .' or 'Finally, let me reiterate my main points . . .' they will listen more carefully.

Concluding pitfalls

- Saying 'And finally . . .' more than once
- Raising new issues during the summary
- Rushing to keep within time. Cut the content, not the introduction or conclusion. These are the most important parts
- Failing to provide time for questions
- Ending on a weak 'Thank you', 'I think that's all I have to say' or 'I can't think of anything else'.

Invent an introduction and title

The title of your presentation is often the first contact you have with your audience, and it may be your last, if it is uninspiring. The trick is to encapsulate the message, but keep it brief and arouse interest.

For example, **'Forcing Your Butterflies to Fly in Formation – presentations for success'**. This title makes the content clear, whilst indicating to the audience that nervousness, as part of public speaking, is common but controllable.

'Nursing Care of Gastro-oesophageal Reflux Disease in Adults' encapsulates the message but is not particularly arousing.

Be sure to keep a pencil and paper with you at all times, as the best ideas seem to spring up at the most unusual moments. My imagination seems to be particularly fertile in the car and during the night. I always have a little hand-held dictating machine to capture my ideas. I rarely remember detail in the morning or at the end of my journey, and I can spend a great deal of time and energy trying to hold information in my mind unnecessarily.

The next step is to create your introduction. This is not the time to bore everyone with a long list of your qualifications and experience. You would not be speaking if you were not considered an expert. You can weave your background in, throughout your presentation, if you need to. If you make a list of four or five features about you or your experience which will help build the credibility of your message, you can drop them in as 'pep-me-ups' (see page 14).

Unless it is a very formal occasion, you do not need to thank the person who has introduced you, the audience for coming, or the group for inviting you. Start straight away with your opening sentence.

This is your best opportunity to grab the audience's attention. Do not waste it by starting with 'Can you hear me at the back?' If they cannot, you will soon know, and anyway you should have checked all your equipment beforehand. The audience will tend to make up their mind about whether to continue to listen to you within the first two to four minutes of your presentation. Clearly, you only have that period of time to get their attention. That is why it is so important to start with something memorable or surprising, a short and interesting quote or an amazing statistic.

For example, instead of opening with 'There are 20 000–30 000 resuscitations every year ...' you could try 'In the time it will take to make this presentation, three people will have endured resuscitation somewhere in this country, whether successful or unsuccessful'.

Introductory pitfalls

- Apologising for anything unless you have hurt someone. Do not ever apologise for your nerves, inexperience or lack of preparation
- Starting with 'Before I begin ...', 'Good morning everybody' or 'Today I'm going to talk about ...' These are tired, old beginnings

- Admitting you are not prepared. If you have not pre-pared, you should not be speaking. If you really have been caught on the hop, do not admit it, give it your best shot and therefore your best chance for success
- Asking about time. 'How much time have I got?' etc. Do not waste precious seconds. These details should be clarified before you get up to speak
- Immediately haranguing members of the audience with questions. It is a good idea to involve the audience as early as possible, but you do not want to alienate them, by making them feel threatened
- Moaning about your difficulties, for example worries about getting to the venue or feeling ill or tired. The audience do not want to be burdened with your prob-lems
- A joke that falls flat. To open with a joke takes real skill and is a risk. Unless you are quite confident that you will be able to handle the situation if it goes wrong, do not take that risk.

You could try starting with one of the following.

1 **A rhetorical question** that will engage the audience straightaway and get them to think. You can control the situation more confidently if you do not ask for a response in words. For example, 'Evidence-based prac-tice – is there a mixture of motives?' or 'Should nurses have spoken out when unexpectedly high numbers of babies died after operations by two surgeons?'. The audience can then answer the question in their own mind.

2 **A quote** which brings your message alive. For example, 'Chance favours the prepared mind', Louis Pasteur. Sometimes speakers are tempted to use rather lengthy literary quotes, which lose the audience. It is better to use short ones, the relevance of which can be seen quickly.

3 **An interesting statistic.** If you do decide to use a statistic, make sure it is from a credible source, not a tabloid newspaper. Round off any numbers to make them memorable. For example, 'Making a poor presenta-tion for 30 minutes to 200 people will waste over four days', rather than 4.1875 days or 6030 minutes.

4 **A story or anecdote.** People, young and old, love stories about other people, success and personal events. Those in health care tend to be particularly interested in

others. You can watch listeners settle down with their ears pinned back when you start with 'Last Thursday I was driving to work when . . .' or 'I'd like to tell you about something that happened . . .'.

5 **A reference to history.** For example, 'On 14 September 1886 the typewriter ribbon was patented' or 'On 22 May 1947 the first ballistic missile was fired'.

6 **Dramatic start.** A paediatric colleague once began a presentation on childhood injury by walking up onto the podium, carrying a doll swaddled in a blanket in her arms. After standing for several minutes crooning to the 'baby', she shook it violently and threw it to the floor. Having grabbed our attention, she proceeded to talk to us about child protection issues.

During the introduction it is important to clearly identify what you are going to be talking about, how you are going to be talking about it, for example dialogue with the audience or questions at the end, etc., and why it will be of interest to the audience.

The WAM factor is crucial. What About Me? Listeners need to be clear about how they will benefit from listening to you. If there seem to be no direct benefits, they will lose interest quickly.

It is important to remember that juries tend to recall only 60 per cent of what they hear. No matter how hard they try to concentrate, the case is not about them. Try to talk to the self-interest of your audience at all times. You should then get your message across.

> **WAM**
> **W**hat
> **A**bout
> **M**e?
> factor

Build the body

From the moment you knew about this presentation, you will have been collecting information together in your document wallet. By writing each idea on a separate index card, you can arrange them into three to five columns of related ideas. Try various arrangements until you find the most powerful one. Make sure you include only what is important or helpful for the audience. Constantly refer to your 'end', to maintain focus.

Remember the story of the man on Tower Bridge, who was poised ready to leap to his death in the River Thames. A policeman, a paramedic and a parson were all called to the scene to reason with him. They begged him to consider

> The secret of being a bore is to tell everything
>
> *Voltaire*

all the reasons to go on living, but with no success. Suddenly a vagrant appeared behind the man and said, 'You don't want to jump into that freezing and smelly water, it's revolting!'. With that, the would-be suicide promptly climbed back over the rail.

This story should remind you to consider the WAM factor (What About Me?) at every step. To get other people to listen to your ideas, you must look at things from their angle.

Stick to the KISS principle (Keep It Short and Simple). Use short words and short sentences. You cannot go wrong if you aim your presentation at a group of reasonably intelligent 13-year-olds. If the audience have to struggle to understand any words or concepts, they are likely to give up. When Abraham Lincoln made the Gettysburg Address, he used very few words longer than five letters. One of the best presentations I have given followed a brief by the course leader to use words of no more than two syllables. Get rid of any clichés and use exciting descriptive words that paint pictures in the minds of the audience. You can never be too clear, so avoid using a big word when a little one will do. It is surprising how many people use the word 'utilize' in place of the word 'use'.

Use pronouns to involve your audience, such as 'we', 'us', and especially, 'you'. 'You' is reputed to be the most popular word in the English language. Instead of saying 'The benefits are ...' you will get a better response from 'This is how your care will improve ...' or 'This is how you will benefit ...'.

Beware of TLAs (Three Letter Abbreviations). As health care professionals we are often guilty of resorting to our exclusive professional jargon. We are all aware of the problems which can result when communicating with patients and relatives. However, just as much confusion can arise within, and between, professions. More importantly, jargon signals that your presentation is what you want to say rather than what the audience needs to hear.

Most people are not able to retain more than seven key points, but even seven is significant. To play safe, it is often better to cover no more than three to five main points. Once you have done all your research, it is tempting to squash everything you know into the session, in an attempt to avoid waste. However, the minds of the audience will not be able to absorb it. If the content does not lead

---

KISS
Keep
It
Short
and
Simple

Avoid TLAs
Three
Letter
Abbreviations

directly or indirectly to the audience's 'end', leave it out. Use the minimum number of facts, views and opinions to convey the message. Successful negotiators use fewer reasons per argument, sticking rigorously to the strongest reason, and occasionally reaching for something equally strong to support it.

Some speakers will claim their presentation must be an exception to the KISS (Keep It Short and Simple) principle, as their subject is just too complex. If the bible can cover the whole of creation in 600 words, it is likely that you can cover your area in fewer.

Certainly the body of your presentation will need to be divided into chunks. The average attention span of a British member of the audience is thirteen minutes, and North American spans will often be as short as eight minutes, reflecting commercial breaks on television (Gilchrist and Davies, 1996).

Exercise

What do the following abbreviations mean to you?

1 FBC
2 PID.

Answers

1 Fluid Balance Chart or Full Blood Count
2 Pelvic Inflammatory Disease or Prolapsed Intravertebral Disc.

Natural and logical linking of ideas or components is essential. Moving smoothly from point to point is an important skill to learn, to keep listeners with you. Transitions might include:

> *My next point is . . .*
> *This leads me to . . .*
> *After . . . comes . . .*
> *The fourth idea is . . .*

When dealing with data, facts and figures, pick the first, largest, newest, latest or smallest. If the audience need all the information, make it available in a handout for them afterwards. It is your job to take the audience behind the numbers. Tell them what the figures mean, which ones point to a trend and which ones point nowhere. The secret of presenting numbers is to identify the dead ones, bring the others to life and keep summarizing. Do not risk boring the audience to death.

Lists of three are excellent for retention. If you make use of alliteration too, retention is even greater. You can make use of lists of three by using three arguments, answers or examples to make your point. For example, fair, fat and forty, or airway, breathing and circulation.

Remember to use only up-to-date, credible and reliable sources. Nurses, particularly, are sometimes accused of forgetting to support their statements with evidence.

Pop in pep-me-ups

Throughout your presentation you need to throw in pep-me-ups. These can be anecdotes, interesting visuals or bits of humour. There is a tendency among inexperienced speakers to describe new or complex ideas from their own personal point of view, and to use examples and pictures that are meaningful to them. Go back to those questions you asked before starting to prepare. Who will be in the audience? What is their background? What will their interests and experiences be?

It is not just children who love a good story. Quantities of facts, without any application, can get very tedious. However, gratuitous stories can be destructive to your 'end'. It is essential that any story, no matter how exciting, is tied directly to the point being made.

When you have decided to tell a story, ask yourself the following questions. What did it smell, taste, feel, sound and look like? Keep it short. As one colleague said, 'Don't tell me where you bought the matches, just tell me how big the fire was'. Where possible, relate your own experiences which make stories more immediate, more credible and easier to remember.

Remember that one of the most interesting things to people is glorified, refined gossip. Tell the audience stories of two people you have known and why one failed and the other succeeded. They will listen and learn.

If you use a direct quote as a pep-me-up, read it from a card or page, so that the audience can see you reading it. If

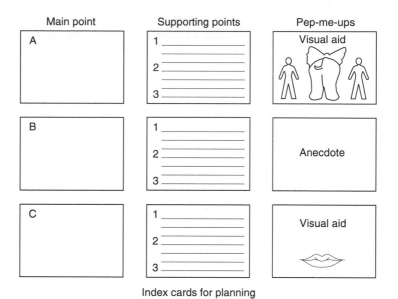

Figure 2.2 Example of index cards with main points on the left, supporting points in the centre and ideas of pep-me-ups and visual aids on the right.

you make it clear who you are quoting and where you got it from, you can add authority to your message.

In order to keep the main body of my presentation structured and focused, I write my three to five main points on separate index cards. I then write the supporting points on another card and place them under the main point cards. I complete this period of preparation by adding a final card outlining pep-me-ups and ideas for visual aids (Figure 2.2).

> Brevity is the best recommendation of any speech
>
> *Cicero*

Vitalize visual aids

Work at the Wharton Centre for Applied Research at the University of Pennsylvania showed that in meetings where decisions are made, visual aids significantly influence those decisions. However, visual aids should be just that, visible and aids. How many times have you heard a speaker apologize for the clarity of a slide? There is no excuse, if it is not clear it should not be shown.

With the advent of fancy computer programmes, some untrained presenters get carried away with the presentation of their slides or overhead transparencies. Sadly, audiences will often leave such presentations very impressed with the 'look' of the visual aids, but with no change in their understanding or opinion. Many of us have access to experts in the audio-visual departments of our hospitals and organizations, but we do not take advantage of them. There are certainly a number of principles to be followed:

- One basic point per visual
- Restrict the number of words to six across, and lines to six down
- Legibility, neatness and correct spelling are essential
- Present figures as diagrams or graphs
- Familiarize yourself with any equipment
- Rehearse with visual aids
- For a speech of twenty minutes, plan no more than eight visual aids
- Show visual aids only when you are talking about them.

Do not dismiss some of the more easily and cheaply produced visual aids. Use what is appropriate for the venue. Slides for an informal group of five people are probably inappropriate, as is a flip chart for 500. (See Handling visual and mechanical aids, Chapter 3.)

There are, of course, non mechanical ways of helping an audience to visualize your message. If I asked you to explain the difference between a million and a trillion dollars, what would you say? When President Reagan talked about his first budget, he said 'A few weeks ago I called such a figure, a trillion dollars, incomprehensible. I've been trying to think of a way to illustrate how big it really is. The best I could come up with is to say that a stack of $1000 bills in your hand, only four inches high, would make you a millionaire. A trillion dollars would be a stack of $1000 bills, seventy-six miles high'.

Tailor for the audience

Look for the WAM factor (What About Me?). By identifying what will motivate members of your audience to listen to what you have to say, you can focus effectively during the first few moments of your presentation. Listeners need to know what is in it for them.

Speakers occasionally make the mistake of preparing a presentation to be given to a number of different groups, without considering how to change the focus in line with what is required by each unique collection of people. I have heard a presentation given to a group of cardiothoracic surgeons and then delivered, unchanged, to a hospital League of Friends, composed of non-clinical people. The presenter was disappointed when the League did not express an interest in providing financial support for a new venture. Had she considered the WAM factor, she would probably have been more successful.

If you are able to influence how long to speak for, the optimum length of time is probably around twenty minutes. Remember that it is better to finish before the end of your time slot, rather than run over time. Once you go over your allocated time, audience members start to fidget and wonder whether the whole programme will run late. Continuing to run over time is one of the easiest ways to antagonize your audience. It is also annoying for anyone speaking after you, as they then have to shorten their own presentation to avoid running late themselves. No matter how tempting, it is arrogant to assume that what you have to say is more important than anyone else's material.

Plan your timings on the premise that your performance on the day will take 25–50 per cent longer than any rehearsal. Be prepared to make cuts if your time is short, but do not cut the conclusion or introduction. An easy way to accomplish this is to colour code your presentation into three sections: must know, should know and could know. Choose a different coloured pen for each section, so you know immediately which section to cut if you need to.

Once you think you have finished writing your presentation, tailor it. The chances are it is too long. I usually have to cut my own presentations in half and take three things out. Then imagine you are in the audience listening to yourself. Remind yourself of who will be listening. Will you cover what they expect to be covered? Make sure you have not included any sexist, doctorist, nursist or racist comments. These will be sure to alienate someone in the audience. Once one person is alienated, others will follow. If you watch carefully, you can see one individual take offence and, shortly afterwards, their body language is mirrored by several others around them. If in doubt, leave it out.

Are there any issues to avoid? If so, why? I remember talking to a group of nurses from Gloucestershire, just after Rosemary West was convicted, who responded to a gentle quip about murder, with stony silence. Speakers need to be sensitive to wider issues than health and conventional politically correct comments.

Make notes

There are a number of differing views about the use of notes during presentations. I rarely stand up to speak without notes. For me, it is like walking a tightrope without a safety net. Without notes, whilst everything is going well, people are fleetingly impressed, but if something goes wrong, it can be very uncomfortable for everyone.

My mind often goes blank whilst giving a presentation, and I can recover my direction by referring to well-prepared notes. These can be used so skilfully that audiences remain unaware of them. There are a number of methods including three inch by five inch index cards, A4 sheets of paper in plastic sleeves to prevent rustling, notes on revealing cards for transparencies or transparency frames. There is no best way, you need to choose the most comfortable method for you.

Always make a copy of your notes, as they have a frightening habit of disappearing just when you need them. When using notes:

- Keep them at waist level and to one side
- Make sure they lie flat
- Use stiff paper or cards on one side only
- Remember that pink highlighter is often easier to see than other colours, in darker conditions
- Text should cover only the top two-thirds of any page. If you fill cards or pages right to the bottom, you will find your chin sinks further and further into your chest, which makes eye contact and adequate voice projection almost impossible
- Times New Roman Type is easiest to read, although handwriting may be even clearer. Use upper and lower case, as you pick up words by scanning the ascenders and descenders, that is, the stalks going above the line and the tails below
- Block capitals are difficult to read quickly. Without the stalks and tails of lower case letters, it takes longer to recognize letters and words
- Number the pages so if they are dropped you can put them back in order. Tying them together with a treasury tag will also protect them from muddle
- Use only key words, with colour and symbols. The eye can only take in four words at a time
- Rehearse with your notes. Much of the memory jogging

comes from the shape of the text rather than individual words. If you make a fresh set of notes just before the presentation, they will not be familiar to you

● Read quotes or statistics from your notes, to make sure they are accurate.

Winston Churchill was renowned for his ability to speak eloquently, and at length, without notes. However, on one memorable occasion, whilst making a crucial speech, his mind went blank and he was unable to recover his composure. From that day he always carried notes with him, although he was never seen to use them. When asked about this habit, he retorted 'I carry fire insurance, but I don't expect my house to burn down'.

When a presenter reads from a full script, it is almost always frustrating for the audience. We can read at approximately 500 words per minute, whereas we can only speak at around 100. By reading from a script you lose spontaneity and audience interaction. Your head will be bowed, making eye contact impossible, voice projection difficult and it is easy to lose your place in the notes. Occasionally, reading a script is unavoidable, for example when reading a press release. On these occasions, make sure you write the script so that it sounds natural when read. You will find letters of at least 14 font, covering only the top two-thirds of the page, easiest to read.

Remember that during verbal communication, the communicator generally uses one- to two-syllable words, simple sentences and pauses at the end of thoughts. Written communication uses two-, three- and four-syllable words, complex sentences and pauses at punctuation marks.

John Hilton, a BBC broadcaster prior to World War Two, suggested using 'speaking style even when it is necessary to read. To read as if you were talking, you first write as if you were talking. What you have on the paper in front of you must be talk stuff, not book stuff'.

Rehearse

There is no alternative to rehearsal. You need to rehearse until the content of your presentation is second nature. Say it aloud when you are alone, in front of people when you have the opportunity, and take it seriously. Practise as if you were performing, but do not try to learn the script off by heart. The audience will see you trying to remember words through your eye movements. Also, memorizing will get in the way of your flow. You will find yourself searching your memory for words rather than concentrating on making your point effectively to the audience. You need to focus on communicating ideas, not phraseology. Memorizing word for word imprisons your thoughts rather than sets them free.

If you can find people to listen and give you feedback, for example, colleagues, spouse or children, you will always be able to find ways of improving. If you are not able to, you may want to talk to a clock. It has a face and you are able to watch your timing carefully. I practise when I am in the car. I sometimes make an audio tape of myself making the presentation, and then play it while driving. This helps me to familiarize myself with the content, so I can concentrate on delivery when I have a rehearsal audience. Lloyd George, when he was a member of a debating society in Wales, often strolled along country lanes talking and gesturing to the trees and fence posts.

If you make an audio tape or, even better, a video tape of yourself, you will be able to hear how your voice really sounds to others. This will cut out distortion through bones and sinuses, which makes the difference between what we hear and what others hear when we talk. Watch or listen to your tape and make a note of things you want to modify. Practise a few more times without taping, but making the modifications you have identified. When you tape yourself again, you should notice improvements. A good rule to follow is to make sure that if you stumble more than once over a word as you rehearse, replace it with another one. One anaesthetist, who speaks internationally, always stumbles over the word 'anaesthetist' when speaking in public. Very few people have noticed that he manages to avoid this word when making presentations.

Rehearsal should take place at the venue, in the clothes you plan to wear, with your visual aids and notes, in real time. There is sometimes a temptation to miss this step and to read your presentation through a few times. This is not enough. Some speakers repeatedly stop part of the way through their presentation and then go back to the beginning. They end up rehearsing the beginning plenty of times, but the ending not at all. Remember that preparation and practice more than compensate for any lack of talent.

Once you have put together your presentation, make sure you have planned ahead and given yourself enough time to put it to one side and return to it after a day or so. A fresh mind spots mistakes, confusing areas and generates new ways of presenting material. This stage, in the past, has allowed me to polish my performance to a real shine.

Remember, the greater your knowledge, the more you need structure and rehearsal.

> **Repetition is the mother of retention**

Preparation to delivery

Once you have put all this hard work into preparing your presentation, do not let anything stand in the way of delivering it. There are only three excuses for not turning up or even being late for a presentation: death, serious illness or critical injury. A cold does not count and neither does a broken bone if it is more than a few days old.

You can plan for other disasters and make sure they are avoided by:

- Having detailed instructions, including a map of how to get to the venue. The best place to get them from is someone at the venue itself. When you are attending an interview or a crucial presentation, it is worth having a dummy run. If you get lost on the day, even if you are not late, you will put yourself under unnecessary pressure
- Being aware of parking arrangements
- Knowing how to get into the venue if you are to arrive after hours
- Getting two contact names and numbers at the venue. That way, if you cannot get hold of one person, you should be able to contact the other
- Carrying a mobile phone. However, always, always remember to switch off mobile phones or pagers before your presentation, or anyone else's. I watched in wonder, when one speaker interrupted his presentation to respond to his mobile phone call. What kind of message do you think he gave to those listening? If you are expecting an important call, arrange for someone else to take the message

- Allowing double the travel time advised. You can always use the extra time for familiarizing yourself with the venue or rehearsal
- Making alternative transport arrangements in case of problems. For example, familiarize yourself with train times if you are driving.

Summary

So, now you know. Preparation begins before you agree to speak. There is no need to rush to the library two weeks before your presentation. As soon as you know what you are to cover, start a presentation file and begin your preparation. Nobody would dream of trying to build a house without a plan. Give some structure to your preparation. If you do not like mine, devise your own, but use it every time, whether you have seven minutes or seven months notice. 'Begin with the end in mind' and then practise, practise, practise.

> **Practise makes perfect and permanent**

References

Covey, S.R. (1989) *The Seven Habits of Highly Effective People*. Simon & Schuster, London.

Gilchrist, D. and Davies, R. (1996) *Winning Presentations*. Gower, London.

3 Handling visual and mechanical aids

Visual aids should be just that, visible and aids. A presenter who attempts to leave a message with their audience without using visual aids, must usually be a superb speaker with a compelling message and spellbinding delivery. However, most of us are not spellbinders. The vast majority of our audiences will have been brought up with the sophisticated visuals of television and will demand high standards of visual aid.

Visual aids should be big, bold and brilliant. If people cannot see your aids, do not use them, as they will be distractions not aids. How many times have you heard a speaker apologize for the clarity of a slide? There is no excuse, if it is not clear it should not be shown. Sophisticated computer programmes have been developed which can produce ornate multicoloured visuals at the press of a button; some untrained presenters get carried away with the presentation of their slides or overhead transparencies. Sadly, such efforts may well get in the way of your message. The audience becomes fascinated by the presentation of the visual aids, and loses the point of your content.

The value of visual material should not be underestimated (see Figure 3.1).

| Visual aids should be big, bold and brilliant |

Why are visual aids so useful?

Visual aids can be used for a number of purposes. They can be used to clarify complex ideas. A picture really is worth a

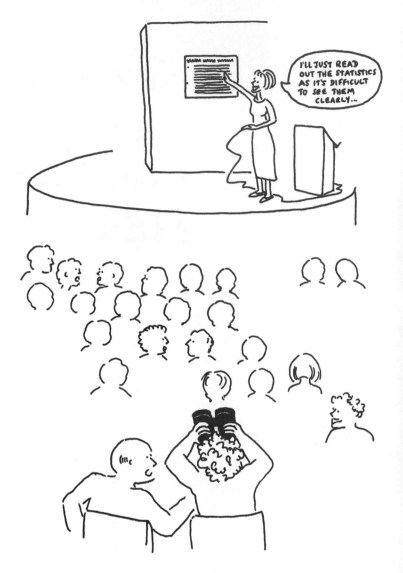

thousand words. Imagine trying to describe what a grade IV pressure sore looks like, in words. Compare that with showing a picture. It is much quicker and much more effective.

Visual aids can be used as notes for the presenter. A number of my colleagues swear that they cannot see notes properly, at the same time as being able to make eye contact and focus on the faces of the audience. They use slides or overhead transparencies as aides-mémoire. If you

People remember 10 per cent of what they read
20 per cent of what they hear
30 per cent of what they see
50–70 per cent of what they see and hear

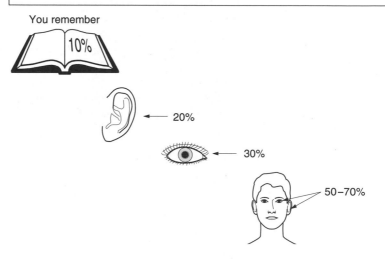

You remember

Figure 3.1 A breakdown showing the proportion of the message remembered by different means.

are going to rely on this system, do make sure you have a back up, in case of mechanical failure.

I find that by starting with a really good transparency, slide or another exciting visual, I can control my nervousness better. I often feel uncomfortable at the beginning of a presentation, with everyone's eyes on me. With just a few moments to acclimatize myself, whilst the audience are concentrating on looking at something other than me, I can find enough confidence to begin.

Visual aids can be used as the pep-me-ups described on page 14. If the audience can only concentrate for thirteen minutes at a time, an interesting picture or diagram can break up dialogue and regain the attention of anyone whose concentration is waning.

What goes wrong?

Be in control of your equipment

Bearing in mind all these good reasons for using high quality aids, do not be tempted to think state-of-the-art support intrinsically improves the presentation. Never take unfamiliar risks with new technology, progress slowly. The first time I used computer generated and projected slides, I worked with an unfamiliar system. Unfortunately, the mouse produced an arrow on the screen, which I could not control and which moved around my slides with what seemed like a mind of its own.

Visual aids must add value to the presentation. They must reinforce, illustrate or explain. Too many can over-power. We have all sat in audiences where speakers stagger onto the podium carrying a stack of transparencies or two carousels of slides. You can almost hear the groans of those present.

There are some basic pitfalls that can be avoided for most forms of visual aid.

Visual aid pitfalls

- Too many words on one visual. Keep It Large and Legible (KILL). If your text were to be mounted on a bill board at the side of the road, those going past in a car at seventy miles per hour should be able to understand the message
- Use of sentences not key points. Start each line with an action word and use the minimum of punctuation.
- Numbers presented without diagrams or graphs. These are boring to look at, and audiences will not bother to even read them, let alone remember them
- Unnecessary logos, names and dates. Speakers will often put their own name or that of their organization, along with the date, in different places on their visuals. This adds no value and just makes the visual busier, taking away from the main message
- Illegibility, untidiness and misspelling. Remember, if you feel the urge to apologize for a visual, do not use it
- Leaving insufficient time to produce aids. If you want to have slides made up, medical illustration departments and commercial companies will often need at least five working days to produce your work, even if you have made the slides on a computer
- Using photocopied or typed text, which is boring to look at and illegible beyond the second row
- Using numerous different type faces. Limit yourself to one or two typefaces and do not overuse italics
- Not making time to rehearse with aids. This becomes obvious when presenters are continually looking over their shoulder to check their aid. It leaks a negative

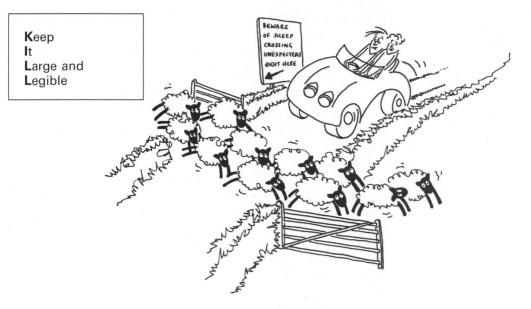

Keep
It
Large and
Legible

message about your concern for the audience, and interferes with eye contact. Once you turn your back to those listening, they will have difficulty hearing

- Reading from the screen. Keep your shoulders orientated toward the audience at all times, and try to maintain eye contact as much of the time as possible.

Tips

NEVER:
- Use photocopied or typed text
- Read from the screen

AVOID:
- Too many words on one visual
- Using sentences
- Numbers without diagrams
- Too much colour and too many different fonts

ALWAYS:
- Use key words
- Check material for spelling and legibility
- Allow time for good quality visual aids to be produced
- Rehearse with the equipment

Colour and fonts

No colour or too much colour may be a problem. Be careful about using red and green for text, as some of the audience may be colour blind. The initial attention span per visual aid averages eight seconds. This increases to eleven seconds as colour is added. Photo backgrounds on visuals increase attention span initially to sixteen seconds per visual. However, two to three colours are enough, except when using photographs or video of course. Apparently men prefer and remember violet, dark blue, olive green and yellow. Women have the best recall when dark blue is used, followed by olive green, yellow and red. However, blue seems to be the favourite colour of most people.

When choosing fonts for text, choose Helvetica, Arial or another sans serif bold print, which is easier to read on a screen, particularly from a distance or if the equipment is slightly out of focus. Sans serif does not have the little feet which connect letters the way serif does. The connections make it easier to read books or newsprint, but not words on a screen. *Choose 26–30 font size for maximum visibility*.

Using charts and graphs

Good graphics give the viewer the greatest number of ideas in the shortest time, with the least ink, in the smallest space. Limit the data you present to the essential. Too much will overface the audience and they will lose interest. If you are using pie charts, make sure your 'slices of pie' accurately represent the figures they are supposed to. Make sure all numbers and calculations are correct. When audiences pick up inconsistencies, they tend to focus on them and lose the thread of the presentation. The presenter will also lose credibility; if the data is inaccurate, what about the rest of the information? Some presenters use three-dimensional bar charts, which might look more exciting, but are more difficult to read. There are other ways of making such charts more interesting.

Graphically represented data must speak for itself. If you have to interpret it for the audience, it is too complex. Charts and graphs are much more interesting when combined with some interesting graphics (Figure 3.2).

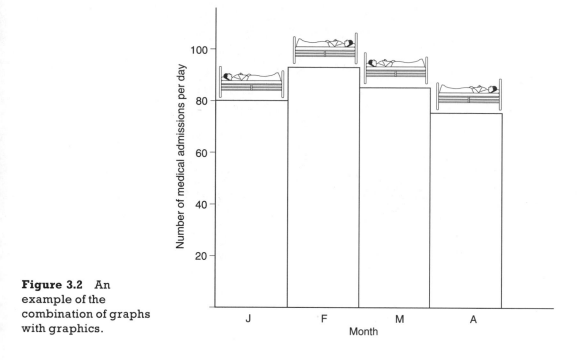

Figure 3.2 An example of the combination of graphs with graphics.

Common forms of visual aid

Overhead projector (OHPs) transparencies

The last decade has seen a dramatic increase in the use of OHPs. In the 1980s it was considered rather amateur to use OHPs as opposed to 35 mm slides. However, pre-senters are starting to realize how much cheaper, more flexible and more easily produced OHPs are. Overhead projector equipment is also easier to manage and less likely to break down.

Another advantage of using an OHP is that it does not require the presenter to dim the lights. This makes a great deal of difference when maintaining eye contact and keeping the audience alert. The machine can produce a large image and is reasonably portable and available. Very professional-looking transparencies can now be produced, particularly if you have access to a colour printer. They can be mounted in frames on which the presenter's notes can be written.

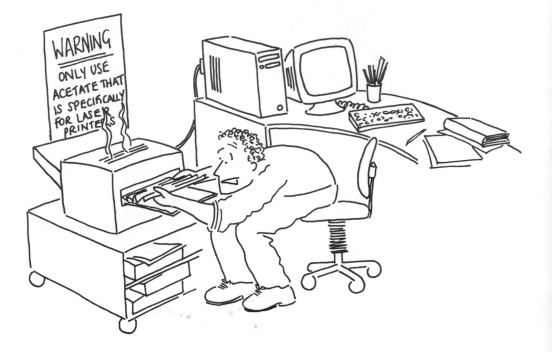

Drawbacks include the requirement for power, occasional breakdown of equipment, noisy fans inside the machine and the problem of the lens blocking some of the audience's view.

If you have a laser printer and want to print transparencies on your own, you can buy a box of blank acetate sheets from a stationery suppliers. You must make sure that you have the correct type of acetate, as the wrong one can melt inside the printer resulting in expensive damage.

Tips for using OHPs

- Good OHPs can be produced without a colour printer, by printing monochrome (black and white) slides and then using OHP pens to incorporate some colour
- Use a horizontal or landscape format, not a mixture. The most natural, eye-pleasing layout is one that has more width than height, that is, landscape (see Figure 3.3)
- Check for readability by standing ten feet away from the transparency when not projected
- Use a beaded screen, not just a plain wall, for maximum

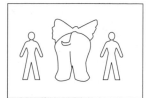

Format: Landscape ✓

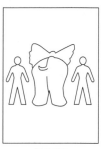

Portrait ✗

Figure 3.3 A demonstration of how format can affect legibility of your OHP.

Figure 3.4 Keystoning.

clarity. The top of the screen should be tilted forward to prevent keystoning (Figure 3.4A). The bottom should be at least four inches from the floor

- To avoid having to switch the machine on and off between transparencies, a white card can be flipped down over the lamp (Figure 3.4B), or a plain piece of paper can be placed in a transparency frame. Let the visual speak and then get rid of it. The rule is 'Use it or lose it', so it is not competing with you
- Pictures can be re-sized on a photocopier, placed on a piece of paper with text and then photocopied onto a transparency
- Avoid projector glare around the edges of your OHPs with masking tape
- Focus the projector by laying a coin or pen on the glass plate. You will then avoid revealing your first visual aid before you are ready
- Stand to the right of the projector from the audience's point of view. They will then be able to look at the visual from left to right, letting their eyes follow on naturally to you when they have finished
- Look at the machine not the screen, unless you are making a really important point. The use of pointers is controversial, some people find them useful, others consider them pretentious
- By placing a piece of card underneath the transparency, you will be able to reveal the contents at your own pace, as well as being able to see what is written
- Instead of using a telescopic or laser pointer, you can lay a pencil or pen on the transparency to draw the audience's attention to particular points
- Have a system for keeping your used and unused transparencies separate during the presentation, to avoid muddle
- If you are able to add information to transparencies while they are on the screen, you can add a sense of action. It is also a sign that you are in control
- If you use water soluble marking pens, you can wipe the transparency off afterwards. However, permanent pens will not smudge or wear as badly with time
- When bulbs blow out, some OHPs have a built in remedy with two bulbs installed. If the first bulb blows, turn the power off, switch to bulb two and then turn the projector on again. Not all OHPs have this facility, so it is essential that you know how to change

a bulb, or how to get hold of someone quickly, who can
- When you arrive early at the venue, approach the technician, get a spare bulb and learn how to install it.

Further tip

Leave visuals up for twice as long as it takes to read from the screen

35 mm slides

Although slides have been the standard aid for formal presentations for years, the culture has started to change. In the past, presenters have used slides badly in the following ways.

Slide pitfalls

- Too many slides for each presentation. For a twenty minute presentation no more than eight slides should be used. Certainly, they should not be changed any more frequently than every 60–90 seconds
- Cardboard slide mounts that get warped and jam easily. Glass mounts may cost more, but they are longer lasting and more reliable
- Busy slides. There should be no more than six words in the title, no more than six lines in total and no more than six words in a line. The font should be a minimum of 18 point, styles should not be mixed and the minimum of punctuation should be used. Do not use all upper or all lower case. Any templates should be simple
- Room not dark enough. To achieve a clear image, the room must be dark enough. Dark backgrounds to the slides with light typeface, work best
- Laser pointers should be used with care. They can be useful to highlight from a distance. However, they should be used sparingly. They are sometimes called nerv-o-meters, as the laser dot jumps around the screen. You can rest your arm on the lectern to keep the dot steady. A number of people sitting in the audience will find these pieces of equipment irritating, so you may want to avoid using them altogether.

Further tips

ALWAYS:
- Number the slides
- Use a hand remote control
- Pause when a new slide appears on screen
- Use a blank slide at the end to avoid unnecessary glare

AVOID:
- Too many slides per presentation
- Cardboard slide mounts that tend to warp
- 'Busy' slides

CAUTION:
- Use laser pointers with care

Tips for slides

- Carousel slide trays are less likely to stick than straight ones
- Number the slides to correspond with the carousel slot number, place them correctly in the carousel and tape the lid down. Do not use paper dots to number, as they can cause the slide to jam in the gate. There are eight ways to load a slide into a carousel and only one of them is right
- Place the projector on a high stand at the back of the room. This will produce the largest possible image and move the projector noise away from you and the listeners. Ask the organizers to unscrew any light bulbs shining on the screen to get the clearest possible image
- If the carousel becomes jammed, make sure the locking ring (the clear top cover) is secure by twisting it clockwise. Then turn the unit over and line up the two matching symbols on the bottom
- Always use a hand remote control to operate slides. If there is not one available, ask for one. These can be purchased at around £150–£200. If you have trouble differentiating between the forward and backward buttons, put a piece of tape on one of them, so you will be able to distinguish between them by touch. Make sure you know where to aim the remote control to advance the slides

- Use a blank slide at the end of your presentation to avoid unnecessary glare for the audience after your last slide
- By using a blank slide at intervals throughout your presentation, your audience will move their necks into a new, lower, and more relaxed position to look at you. This will make them more comfortable and therefore more receptive to your message
- When a slide comes onto the screen, pause for two seconds until the audience has had a chance to focus on it.

Flip chart

The beauty of the flip chart is cost and accessibility. It needs no power and can be prepared in advance. It is adaptable, easy to see and available to refer back to during presentations. However, flip chart sheets are expensive to prepare professionally, cumbersome to carry, will not last long and can look dog-eared.

Tips for flip charts

- Stay on the right-hand side (yours) of the easel and point with the left hand, to avoid getting in the way
- Make sure you have enough clean sheets of paper
- Have appropriate flip chart pens. Water soluble markers, as opposed to permanent markers, do not mark the next pages. You will often find dry white board pens next to flip charts. These work properly for only a few words, before they run out
- Letters need to be at least one inch tall for each fifteen feet to the back row of people. Thick letters in lower case, made with the fat side of the pen, are more easily read. Graph paper makes consistency easier
- Black or blue ink is clearest for text
- Restrict text to the top two-thirds and the right two-thirds of the sheet for visibility
- Mistakes can be rectified with liquid paper (such as Tippex)
- Bulldog clips will hold used pages over the back of the easel
- Pre-scored pages can be torn off neatly
- For fast access to pages, tear off the corner of the previous one or place Post Its® on the edge of the page (Figure 3.5)

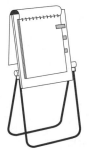

Figure 3.5   Post Its® placed on the edge of the page can give fast access to the required page.

- Light pencil notes can be made on the side of the pages as aides-mémoire for the presenter
- By leaving two blank sheets between pages, or stapling pages together, you will avoid marks from the page before
- A border round your pages can add impact.

Further tips

ALWAYS:
- Stand on the right of the easel
- Use water soluble markers
- Write large enough

TIPS:
- Use Post Its® for easy access to specific pages
- Use black or blue ink for clarity
- Restrict text to top two-thirds of the page
- Use pencil aides-mémoire

Handouts

Handouts can offer an important message to the audience, that they matter enough for the presenter to have prepared material to help them after the presentation. They can be used to highlight important points and give details of references.

Tips for handouts

- Create 15 per cent more than the number you expect to attend
- Tailor them for the specific audience, do not use a handout you designed a year previously for a different group, with different needs
- Wait until the end of your session to hand them out, to avoid unnecessary distractions
- Using the handout as a working document, on which the audience can make notes, sometimes works well
- Put your name, address and contact numbers on the bottom, if you plan to invite people to contact you for further information
- When developing handouts, ask yourself what the audience will want to take away

- Hole punch them, so those present can put them straight into a ring binder.

Further tips

ALWAYS:
- Tailor your handouts to the audience
- Hand out at the end of the session
- Put your contact details on the bottom
- Produce 15 per cent more than expected audience

TIPS:
- Handouts can alternatively be used as a working document throughout the session
- Hole punch handouts for immediate filing and safe keeping

What about three-dimensional objects?

Real objects, such as a model or a piece of equipment, can be powerful as aids. Touch is a very effective learning tool, but not during your presentation. Wait until you have finished to pass anything around. Once the audience have something in their hands, they will tune out from what you are saying.

I remember making a presentation on quality assurance. When talking about quality being a subjective area, we gave out chocolate and asked members of the audience to pass an opinion as to its quality, judging look, taste, feel, etc. We then made the point that quality, like beauty, is in the eye of the beholder. The audience were actively involved right from the start, and everyone loves to get an unexpected present.

I was very impressed by a colleague who demonstrated the vulnerability of the cervical spine when humans are involved in a car crash, by balancing a potato on a straw.

Use imaginative props

Using unusual or unexpected props can engage your audience, add humour and leave a memorable impression. Do make sure that the prop is relevant and will not cause prolonged distraction, though.

General visual aid tips

- Use colour to highlight points rather than decoration, otherwise it will lose its effect
- Always familiarize yourself with the mechanics of using visual aids
- Make sure any flexes are out of the way or taped into a safe place
- Learn how to change bulbs in OHPs and slide projectors. Even better, use a projector with two bulbs
- By standing on the left-hand side of the screen, the audience will be able to read the visual and then let their eyes follow naturally to where you are standing. Make sure you are not obstructing anybody's view
- Make sure you talk to the audience and not to the visuals
- Once you have finished using an aid, remove it from view. However, leave any visuals up for twice as long as it takes you to read them.

Video

When used appropriately, well made video tapes can be very powerful and dramatic. Although it is tempting to leave the showing of video tapes to the control of audio-visual technicians, you are courting disaster. You will need an appropriately sized television screen, tuned into the right channel, with the tape set at the right place.

Audience size	Monitor size
Under 10	19 inches
11–25	25 inches
26–75	4–6 feet

Double check that your video is in the right format and system for the venue. Also remember that every time a video is copied, it loses 12 per cent resolution, so use an original where possible, not a copy.

Use video clips sparingly. Anything more than short clips can be boring and will risk losing the attention of the audience.

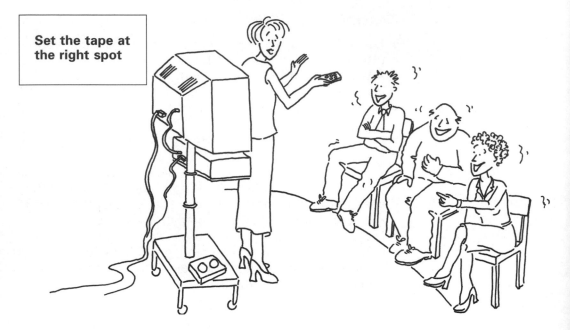

Set the tape at the right spot

Video tips

- Check equipment beforehand, which will save time and embarrassment later
- Pre-set volumes, by setting and then sitting on the back row, to check levels
- Check quality of the picture in the same way
- Always cue your videos before using them
- Always carry a spare tape.

Further tips

ALWAYS:
- Check equipment
- Pre-set volumes to allow good reception in the back rows
- Carry a spare tape

LCD panels and projectors

Liquid Crystal Display projectors are fast replacing slides. When connected to the video port of a computer, they let you project images onto a blank wall or screen. When combined with a laptop computer, they are easy to use, and fairly easy to transport.

LCD panels are designed for use with OHPs. However, for good quality images, the OHP should produce a standard measure of light of no less than 400 lumens. The panel is flat and about the depth of a laptop computer, weighing about seven pounds.

LCD projectors are self-contained units which are much heavier than the panel, although they have everything you need in one place and produce higher quality images.

Before you demonstrate your proficiency with this equipment publicly, make sure you really know what you are doing. They say it takes ten minutes to learn how to remove an appendix, but four years to learn what to do if something goes wrong.

Microphones

At the age of eight years old, I had my first disaster with a microphone. I had taken the part of a Dutch girl and had rehearsed for weeks to be in the Vacation Club Show. My mother and grandmother had convinced me that I could be destined for stardom, as they were pioneers of the Positive Virtual Reality theory. However, I had never actually used a microphone before. As I opened my mouth, I also yanked the microphone towards me, and the resulting noise sounded physiological. Sadly, I was so put off by this unexpected interruption, that I missed every note thereafter and rushed from the stage sobbing. I learned a number of lessons in life that night, not least of which concerns mechanical aids.

Always familiarize yourself with any equipment before a performance, not in front of the audience. If you do not bother to sort everything out beforehand, it can be very difficult to do so with all eyes on you, the audience will become bored and lose interest before you start and the message – amateur – will be loud and clear. You can use the opportunity to check how to turn the switches on and off and to check the volume required. Then, if problems do arise and the equipment becomes a distraction, you can turn it off.

Use a microphone only when necessary, as so many things can, and do, go wrong. If your voice carries well you may think you do not need a microphone. Remember though, that the venue will be full of people, and people absorb sound. If in doubt, at least prepare to use one. It can certainly help whenever you address more than fifty people at a time.

The clip-on microphone is excellent for the inexperienced and those who like to move around. However, it is important to practise clipping it onto your clothes near your second shirt button, about two inches down from your collar, without trembling hands, in front of an audience. Do remember to remove it when you have finished. There are some horror stories circulating about individuals who have rushed to use the toilet afterwards, only to have their ablutions transmitted through loudspeakers in the lecture hall.

Tips

- Familiarize yourself with any equipment before a presentation
- Use a microphone only when necessary
- The clip-on microphone is excellent for the inexperienced

A unidirectional microphone, one which picks up input from a single direction, is often attached to the podium. Your voice will sound best when your mouth is between four and eight inches from the head of the microphone. When using the fixed microphone, practise having it at an appropriate distance from your mouth and at the correct height. Avoid any violent movements and remember that no two microphones are the same, so rehearsal is essential.

If you are using a portable hand-held microphone, hold it just under your mouth like an ice cream cone, and direct your mouth to the farthest corner of the room.

Feedback can sometimes be an embarrassing and annoying problem. This shrill, whistling noise often results from the microphone getting too close to the speakers. If you are walking and talking, stay clear of the speakers. Turn your head if you need to cough, and do not cough into the microphone.

Summary

Effective use of the equipment associated with giving presentations boils down to familiarity. It is essential to build your rehearsal around them. You are asking for trouble by waiting until the morning of the presentation to try to assimilate your content with visual and mechanical aids. Remember the short time you have to create an impression. If you use this time up by stumbling around, trying to dim the lights or get the OHP working, what kind of impression do you think you will create?

Sometimes, there will be a mechanical failure. Plan ahead. What could go wrong, and what will you do if it does? By handling a difficult situation well, you can sometimes create an even more positive impression of yourself.

It ain't what you do, it's the way that you do it

Fun Boy Three and Bananarama

4 Dressing for success

Does your appearance affect the way people perceive you?

The answer is a definite 'Yes'. It may seem unfair, but people are influenced by the way you look. Children as young as two or three months look, respond and smile at some faces more than others.

Those people with childlike faces will often find that others warm to them. Recent research at the University of St Andrews has shown that 'infantile signals' of small noses, full lips, big eyes, small chin and high cheekbones, stir up people's protective instincts. However, such signals can also mean that others will not take you seriously. More mature features, like bigger noses and prominent jaws, may encourage others to consider you as more of an equal. They may be more influenced by you, if not so friendly.

Grey hair is often seen as distinguished in men, although it is considered less appealing in women. Tall and slim people are often judged to be more competent, although thin men may be considered wimpy (Quilliam, 1997).

This prejudice could seem very discouraging, particularly when we consider that we may have only a few seconds to create an impression. However, do not despair. There are so many ways of 'adjusting' our natural look, with posture, clothes, make up and exercise. Psychologists have found that attractive people are more persuasive than unattractive people. However, anyone can cultivate attractiveness, through good grooming and a professional approach.

Health care professionals do not enjoy a good reputation for selling themselves. To sell ourselves effectively, we need to pay attention to our packaging and encourage people to look inside. Many of us try to shirk responsibility by claiming that it is all down to 'charisma'. Charisma can be defined as special, magnetic charm or appeal that allows someone to attain the devotion of large numbers of people. I am of the firm belief that you can learn the skills required to be charismatic. Whether we like it or not, our outward physical appearance is an important factor, and our most valuable visual aid.

Exercise

What did you wear the last time you wanted to make a positive impression at work?

Why did you choose that?

In every election this century in the USA, the taller candidate won (with the exception of one, Jimmy Carter). It is said that Michael Dukakis' failure to win in 1988 was due, in part, to his refusal to wear shoulder pads. What you choose to wear tells the audience about two things:

1 your perception of yourself
2 your perception of the audience.

You can compliment the audience by showing them you have made the effort to dress appropriately. You need to look the part. That means creating an appearance associated with authority, expertise or whatever it is you intend to project. It is not about trying to be someone else, but about developing yourself.

Choosing clothes

You do not need to spend a fortune on clothes to dress appropriately. However, you may need to invest some money, and a certain amount of time and effort. I acquire a number of my outfits for making presentations second hand, so that I can afford better quality. Although I speak quite frequently in public, I usually have only one or two suits I wear alternately for a year. When choosing clothes, stay focused. Be very clear about the message you want to convey to the audience. If you want to appear professional, competent, confident and smart, you need to steer clear of trendy, sexy or 'mumsy' outfits.

Colours

To make sure you get the most you can from different combinations, first select a colour scheme. Unless you have no money and some very expensive clothes, it may be best to ignore what you already own, and choose a neutral base colour that suits you. If you then select medium-weight fabrics, you can wear the clothes all year round. You should spend as much as you can afford for quality, to make sure you get the best value for money.

It can be tempting to choose fashionable and bright colours. Resist this temptation if you can. Obviously such choices can date quickly. Bright colours are usually acceptable for large audiences of 500 people or more. For smaller audiences your clothes can start to outshine the message you are trying to convey. You will find that darker colours are associated with power. Yellow conveys a message of 'like me' and 'I'm not threatening'. Avoid fabrics with a large printed design.

A suit or a blouse in a rich, warm colour can serve as camouflage for those who feel uncomfortable about blushing.

Appearance pitfalls

- Forgetting to consider how you look from the back. Always check how you look in a full-length mirror and get an objective opinion. Do not wait until the day of your presentation to do this
- Unbuttoned jacket. The audience can see your waist, chest or abdomen, which may be a distraction. By doing up your jacket you will look more formal and prepared
- Showing too much skin. The more skin you show, the less authority you will retain
- Badly fitting clothes. The wrong size, too large, small, short or long can be very noticeable and distracting. For those women who are not sure about skirt length, it should probably be no shorter than one inch above the knee

- Gimmicky ties, shirts, socks, or stockings. These will label you as lightweight straight away, which may result in a reluctance to take you seriously
- High heeled shoes. Your posture tends to look awkward and you increase the risk of overbalancing
- Bare legs for women, no matter how hot, are unacceptable
- Heavy fragrances can be very off-putting
- Poorly maintained shoes. These will be visible to the audience, particularly if you are up on a stage. Be particularly mindful of the back of your heel, where many people develop worn patches from driving a car
- Dirty clothes and hair
- Jangling or reflective jewellery or objects in your pocket
- Tinted prescription glasses make it difficult for listeners to get good eye contact from you
- Long, obviously polished nails, particularly on clinicians, can undermine your message
- A change of hair style or colour the day before a presentation. If you do not like it, you will be self-conscious, and it will show.

Tips for dressing successfully

Women:

- A skirted suit is always safe, although a smart trouser suit or matching jacket and skirt is often fine
- Plain court shoes in a darker colour than your hemline, with a medium-sized heel, should be carefully maintained
- Neutral stockings of 15–20 denier in the winter and 7 denier in the summer. Always carry at least one extra pair
- Suitable make up. Even if you do not usually wear make up, you should when making a presentation. Once you have practised, it will only take 10 minutes to apply some blusher, mascara and lipstick. This will give some definition to your eyes and mouth
- Smart, chunky earrings work well, but dangly ones do not.

Men:

- A suit is best, although co-ordinating jacket and trousers are acceptable in less formal settings. You should look for the darkest neutral colour that suits you. Always do the jacket up before taking the floor

- Ties should reach to the waistband of your trousers, not above or below. Always carry an extra tie in case of accidents. I remember attending the Nurse of the Year awards in 1986. As I leaned over the table to take my seat, the tie on my blouse trailed through a mound of avocado dip. For the rest of the lunch I looked as though I had blown my nose on the front of my shirt
- Never wear a pocket handkerchief to match your tie. It looks dated and lightweight
- The waistband of your trousers should rest against your navel
- A good quality belt is worth investing in.
- Five-eighths of your shirt cuff should show beneath your jacket sleeve, for those of you who are striving for perfection
- Socks should be the same colour as your suit or trousers.

Exercise

Imagine a scale of 0–10: 0 should represent you in your underwear and 10 in evening dress. When making a presentation you should probably aim for about 7 on the scale, and certainly one point above the level at which you expect the audience to dress.

One expert in personal presentation once told me that if an outfit is suitable to go out in for the evening, it is probably not suitable for a presentation during the day.

Summary

Perhaps there is some truth in the saying that 'You are what you wear'. In Chapter 6, 'Getting up there', we will explore how long it takes to create an impression. The audience will have made up its mind whether to carry on listening to you within the first couple of minutes. Much of that time you will not even have started to talk, and your appearance will be very important. It is easy to shrug your shoulders and say, 'They must take me as they find me'; if they do not find you pleasing to look at, they will not bother finding you at all. It might seem unfair, but it is a fact of life. You do not need to look like Tom Cruise or Helena Bonham-Carter, but you do need to look well turned out and appropriately dressed. Women in health care should be particularly aware of how easy it is to encourage negative stereotyping with what you wear.

If you wear the wrong clothes, your audience will find you distracting. No matter how much of an expert you are, poorly fitting or inappropriate clothes will make you look insecure, incompetent and unprofessional.

On a final note, do not adopt a 'stage persona', either with regard to personality or the clothes you wear. People watch you before and after you are on show, and they want to see the same person. They want you to 'walk the talk'.

Reference

Quilliam, S. (1997) *Body Language Secrets*. Thorsons, London.

5 Coping with nerves

Cicero is not alone. The *Book of Lists* indicates that fear of speaking in public is ranked ahead of fear of death:

1 speaking before a group
2 heights
3 insects
4 financial problems
5 deep water
6 sickness
7 death
8 flying
9 loneliness
10 dogs.

Having surveyed hundreds of seminar participants before presentation skills training, I have realized that the greatest need for the vast majority has been to be able to control nerves. We wind ourselves up into 'nervous wrecks'. We predict that something will go wrong when we do a presentation and we think there will be nothing we can do about it when it does. Of course, we forget that it is not what happens that is important, it is how you handle it. When something does go wrong there is an excellent opportunity to handle it with grace and confidence, which can often earn more credibility for us than if the process had progressed without a hitch.

We have a tendency to be unrealistically generous to the audience, by assuming that we will have their undivided attention even before we begin. This, of course, is rarely the case. They are more likely to be thinking about what to have for dinner, what shopping they may need to do or what is going to happen at work tomorrow.

Often our fear is rooted in a fear of imperfection. If you can accept the fact that nobody is perfect and neither are you, you will be able to concentrate on the job in hand. Pre-presentation nerves is a rather selfish affliction and perhaps the best approach is to put all that energy into preparing yourself to give the audience the best possible deal.

Telling yourself not to be nervous is like telling yourself not to breathe. Anyway, some adrenaline heightens perception and concentration. According to Hans Selye (1975), stress is not caused by anything within the body, but rather by the way we think about what is happening to us. Whether you think you can or cannot do something, you tend to be right. Self-fulfilling prophecy in this area can be very powerful (see section 'Positive virtual reality').

Mark Leary, in his book *Understanding Social Anxiety* (Leary, 1983), identifies two factors which will determine how nervous you will feel:

1 your prediction of how well you will perform
2 how important you think the consequences of your performance are.

When you attempt to present your ideas or your position to others verbally, you take a risk and you make yourself vulnerable. If you write something and others disagree or misunderstand, they usually do so away from your physical presence. Thus, you are removed from the moment of rejection. You have, at least, some time and privacy to respond.

What do people fear?

This is different for everyone, but one survey suggests that it includes:

- Negative audience reaction
- Difficult questions
- Under- or over-running the time allotted
- Going blank
- Getting in a muddle
- Making a fool of yourself
- Not achieving colleagues' expectations.

Identifying your fears is the first step to controlling them.

Exercise

'What is the worst thing that could possibly happen when I present?' Then ask yourself: 'What would then happen if that happened?'

For example: Making a fool of myself by answering a question wrongly.

- Everyone would feel embarrassed, including me
- I would blush and stutter
- Some of the audience may stifle a laugh
- I will recover some composure
- I will continue to the end of my presentation
- I will feel proud that I was able to finish my presentation.

What can you do?

Once you have identified your particular fears, you can then start to do something about preparing to handle them. Desberg (1996) suggests a 'stress inoculation' where you immerse yourself in the anxiety-provoking situation gradually and then adapt to it with repeated exposures. The more closely you simulate the actual conditions of the presentation during practise, the more secure you will feel on the day. If you practise in a safe, familiar environment, it will be much more difficult in an unfamiliar and tense situation on the day. An interesting experiment carried out during World War II showed that over 80 per cent of the soldiers tested never fired their guns in combat. We have already explored the importance of rehearsal. This issue underlines the importance of full rehearsal at the venue, with visual aids and with people present.

If you feel self-conscious, stimulate your interest in those present. Who has brown hair? How many have a big nose? What is the commonest suit colour? So often, those attending my seminars will reach the end of their presentation demonstration, heave a sigh of relief and go on about how nervous they were. Of course, in reality, those listening were so engrossed in what they could learn from their colleague, they hardly noticed. It seems that people are much more worried about appearing inadequate than they are about failing to communicate a message.

Relaxation

Carried tension shows, and the audience will pick it up.

Exercise

Clench your fist and talk at the same time, and you will notice that your jaw is clenched, which will change your voice production. Simple relaxation techniques known to many of you can be very effective.

- By yawning you can release your jaw and sound more relaxed. It may be best to try to do this out of the view of your audience who may think you are bored before you start
- blowing out your lips with a 'brrr' like a horse, will achieve a similar effect
- an easy-to-read and gripping novel, saved especially for the occasion when I am particularly tense, works wonders for the couple of hours beforehand
- a favourite of mine is to walk briskly around the building, up and down the stairs or even do a few star jumps in the ladies toilets. I then sit in my seat just before getting up to speak and tense all my muscles for a few seconds, followed by a deliberate period of relaxation. Posture exercises can reduce tension effectively
- isometric exercises are stationary exercises in which one group of muscles work against another. You can press your finger tips together, then press harder and hold it for a few seconds. You will find that these will tend to burn nervous energy.

Exercise

1 Stand against the wall with the back of your head, shoulders, buttocks and heels touching the wall. Balance yourself in this position and relax. Walk away from the wall keeping a sense of length in the spine and head.
2 Sit well back in your chair, making sure that you have as much of your back as possible supported by the back of the chair.

Creative visualization

Exercise

Close your eyes and imagine you are somewhere lovely:

1 stretched out in front of a roaring log fire with a wonderful book, a steaming hot chocolate and a cosy cashmere blanket
2 underneath a shady palm on a sandy beach, sipping a pina colada, with the gentle lapping of waves around you
3 in a bath of fragrant warm oil, with your favourite music in the background, laughing at an excellent joke.

Imagine all the pleasures associated with these scenarios, for example, sights, smells and feelings. My favourite is to imagine pausing outside my own front door at home, to smell a lovely flower, and then to watch myself put the key in the lock, turn the handle and walk into comfort and safety.

Positive virtual reality

Sports psychologists and coaches have been using attitude modification and positive mental imaging for years. Other organizations are developing similar concepts called 'mind set re-engineering'.

At the beginning of this chapter I referred to the power of self-fulfilling prophecy. Anxiety is based on a series of ongoing predictions, which keep escalating until you are trapped in a vicious circle. Whether you say you will be great or you will be awful, you tend to be right. With positive virtual reality, the key to success is to say 'You will be great'.

Imagine yourself stepping up to the power position (see Chapter 6, 'Getting up there') to the deafening sound of applause, amidst admiring faces. On your own face is a radiant smile laced with humility and confidence. Then imagine delivering your closing remarks into the attentive silence, followed by a standing ovation. You may not reach these dizzy heights every time, in reality, but you will at least get closer.

During the moments just before your presentation, use some positive self-talk. 'I'm really glad I'm here. I can't wait to get up there. I'm going to be brilliant. I'm going to really make a difference to the audience. Speaking comes naturally to me'. Try whatever words work for you. Once you start concentrating on the words, there is no capacity in your mind for negative and defeatist messages.

Controlling mounting panic

In the past I have frequently experienced an increasing sense of panic as the moment I am to stand up approaches. I have solved this problem by forcing the logical part of my mind into action. This leaves no space for emotional thoughts. You can try counting back in sevens from 620, or you can run your own internal monologue on what you are doing rather than what you are feeling, for example, I am buttoning up my jacket, I am picking up my notes, I am standing and walking towards the front, etc.

I carry a sharp object with me, such as a key, and when panic starts to mount I close my hand around it. It is difficult not to focus on the physical sensation of pain, thereby blocking out any other thoughts.

Controlling other symptoms

Dry mouth

For some people, this problem can cause difficulty with continuing the presentation. At the very least it can be uncomfortable and embarrassing. It is sensible to avoid salty or sugary food and coffee during the hours beforehand. However, you will have different problems if you drink litres of other fluid instead.

A small, wide-based glass, half filled with still water at room temperature is what you need. Delicate wine glasses, filled to the brim, show your trembling hands and risk spillage. Some presenters claim that iced water constricts your throat. Opera singers avoid milky drinks as they are supposed to increase the production of mucus, which coats the vocal cords and makes the tone less clear. Caffeine-containing drinks should be avoided. Anyone prone to jumpiness can be over-stimulated by tea, coffee or cola.

For those of you who find your top lip sticking to your top teeth when you get dry, try smearing petroleum jelly or lip gloss over the surface of your top front teeth.

Exercise

Picture a large, shiny, yellow, juicy lemon. Imagine you are cutting it in half and then sinking your teeth deep into the fleshy middle.

You can try this when no water is available and you are starting to dry up. I find it works every time. You can achieve a similar effect by biting the side of your tongue and counting to ten or having a pinch of salt available.

Excessive perspiration

Hopefully a heavy duty sports antiperspirant will minimize this problem. However, a number of presenters, particularly men, find their upper lip or forehead can drip with perspiration, which is embarrassing and rather obvious. A well-known neurosurgeon always applies a touch of stick antiperspirant over the offending areas, when being interviewed or making a presentation.

Blushing and a red blotchy neck

Having interviewed over 3000 job applicants during my career, I cannot remember many candidates who did not develop red blotches over their face or neck. They are very common, and of only passing interest if the victim is willing to ignore them. However, if you are very self-conscious, you can make them invisible by wearing a high necked shirt or a scarf around your neck. By wearing red or pink colours you can draw attention away from your blotches. For those people whose blushing severely affects their working and personal lives, an endoscopic transthoracic sympathicotomy is a last resort, where the nerve supply to the cutaneous blood vessels of the face is interrupted. This improves symptoms in nearly 98 per cent of patients (Drott *et al.*, 1988).

A blank mind

My mind usually goes completely blank at least three times during any presentation. This used to fill me with dread. Now I just make sure my notes are accessible, leave a silence whilst I regain my composure and then pick up where I left off. Rarely does anyone notice me struggle. In extreme circumstances, when I can barely remember my name, I ask a member of the audience to recap for me. This will help me assess whether the audience have understood what I have said, as well as helping me to get back on line.

Exercise

Use a home camcorder to video yourself. First of all, talk about your job. Then tape yourself a second time and describe an experience where you were really frightened or you were the centre of attention and loved it . What was the difference? Getting your emotions involved really helps. Finally, watch the video with the sound down and in fast forward mode. You should start to pick up some of your bad habits, and realize that short silences are actually beneficial.

Tips for dealing with nerves

- Avoid carbonated drinks during the hours beforehand. Breaking wind during a presentation does not always go down well with the audience. However, if it occurs remember, it is not what happens, it is how you handle it
- Beta blockers are sometimes used to control symptoms of nervousness. Some find the relief enormous. I did try them for a while, although they did not help me at all. Someone then posed the question, 'At what point do you draw the line? It does seem excessive to pump unnecessary drugs round your body, just to make a presentation.' I have no doubt that there are safer and more effective ways to control symptoms. Some claim that naturally occurring beta blockers found in bananas work for them
- Go to bed at a reasonable hour with something absorbing to read. Fatigue affects the way you feel and the way you appear to others
- Exercise on the morning of your presentation. This will use up some adrenaline and release some endorphins

- Eat a light breakfast to help you avoid light-headedness and prevent your stomach from trying to talk at the same time as you. You will probably find that if you indulge in a full English breakfast with plenty of greasy bacon and fried food, you will feel too lethargic and appear sluggish
- Listen to energizing music with a strong beat and driving rhythm. I find that this puts me in the right frame of mind
- Plan something nice as a reward for after your presentation
- Involve the audience in some kind of activity which will hold their attention, increase their retention and reduce your nervousness, by moving the focus off you.

Further tips

Beat nerves:
- Avoid fizzy drinks (and subsequent wind!)
- Get enough rest the night before
- Exercise before the presentation
- Eat a light breakfast
- Listen to upbeat music
- Plan a reward for yourself

Remember:

- The audience want you to succeed. If you fail you will remind them of their own vulnerability
- You have the knowledge they want
- They do not know you are scared. It does not matter how nervous you are, as long as you cover it up
- You can treat the audience as an individual and imagine you are answering a question.

Exercise

Think back to a seminar or a television programme when someone has begun to struggle and has lost control. How did it make you feel?

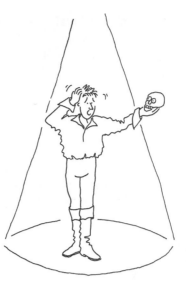

Summary

I am surprised to report that there has not been one recorded death from public-speaking-induced anxiety. Nevertheless, crippling stage fright does not just affect amateurs. Laurence Olivier was suddenly afflicted with it after fifty years on stage, and Barbra Streisand avoided touring for ten years as the result of a blank mind episode. Lloyd George and Disraeli both struggled with nerves in their early years. Some claim that experience reduces anxiety, although research does not support this (Beatty *et al.*, 1989).

I have explored various methods I use for controlling nerves, but you will need to find out what suits you best. Preparation is the key to success. For those of you who are considering drugs or alcohol, think again. By blunting your inhibitions, you will merely fail to notice that your performance is lacking. The result may be slowed reaction time, slurred speech and hazy memory, all adding up to reduced mental agility.

One last suggestion. For situations of extreme pressure, you may want to resort to imagining the audience in a vulnerable position themselves. What about imagining them on commodes, having torrential diarrhoea?

Remember:

Compared with eternity, making a presentation is small fry.

References

Beatty, M.J., Balfantz, G.L., Kuwabara, A.Y. (1989) Trait-like qualities of selected variables assumed to be transient causes of performance state anxiety. *Communication Education*, 38: 277–289.

Desberg, P. (1996) *No More Butterflies*. New Harbinger Publications, Oakland, CA.

Drott, C., Claes, G., Olsson-Rex, L. *et al.* (1998) Successful treatment of facial blushing by endoscopic transthoracic sympathicotomy. *British Journal of Dermatology*, 138 (4): 639–643.

Leary, M. (1983) *Understanding Social Anxiety: Social, Personality and Clinical Perspectives*. Sage Publications, Beverley Hills, Ca.

Selye, H. (1975) *Stress Without Distress*. Cygnet Books, New York.

6 Getting up there

You can't plough a field by turning it over in your mind

Starting rituals establish confidence

For the majority of inexperienced and experienced speakers, walking to the front of a group or climbing onto a stage is the most stressful part of public speaking. Once the presenter has got over the initial anxiety of starting off, they tend to settle down and even enjoy themselves. I have found a 'starting ritual' invaluable in these circumstances. I start every presentation in the same way, so I focus on the ritual, rather than on my anxiety about people watching me or on the 'what ifs?'. This is the path my starting ritual follows:

1 an hour before the presentation, I will take measures to use some of my circulating adrenaline by having a brisk walk around the block or, in extreme cases, running up and down stairs. During this exercise I will think back to some of the successes I have had in my professional life

2 I will make sure that I am confident about the mechanics supporting the session by checking any piece of equipment I may have to use that could go wrong, for example, light dimmers, slide projector, video or microphone (see Chapter 3, 'Handling visual and mechanical aids')

3 for twenty minutes or so beforehand I use an exercise popular with sports people, and imagine myself being a huge success and finishing my presentation to a standing ovation. I repeat to myself 'I know what I'm talking about and I'm pleased I've got the chance to say it'. I will visit the toilet, look in the mirror and say 'I am the best speaker that could have been asked to talk about this today, to this group'

4 for the final few minutes, I will sit in the audience and force my brain into some useless, but logical activity,

such as counting backwards from 372 in 5s. That way my mind does not have time to worry about going blank or anything else that might go wrong

5 as soon as I am invited up to speak, I put a delighted expression on my face, as though there is no place in the world I would rather be. I fix my eyes on a spot on the floor where I am heading, and walk slowly over with as much confidence and grace as possible

6 I place my notes on a table or lectern, look at the audience, make eye contact with two or three members, smile, pause and then start.

Further tips

A pause is a positive tool not a negative action:

- It allows time for the audience to quieten
- Enables you to gather your thoughts
- Gives a message of confidence
- Focuses audience attention

The pause before you speak serves three purposes: it gives time for the audience to quiet down; it gives you a moment to gather yourself; and it signifies a prepared and confident speaker.

Every time I go through this ritual, I am amazed at the confidence I can harness with positive virtual reality (see Chapter 5, 'Coping with nerves').

Body language

The role of body language in communication has increased in profile over the 1990s, although there are differing views about the significance of this non-verbal communication. Albert Mehrabian, professor of psychology at the University of California, has calculated that only about 7 per cent of understanding derives from what is actually said, 38 per cent coming from the tone of voice and 55 per cent from non-verbal cues (Mehrabian, 1972).

Harvard psychologists developed a series of tests in which men and women watched silent film clips of people talking, and were asked to guess what was happening by reading body language and expressions.

Seven keys to success:

- **Body language**
- **Posture**
- **Eye contact**
- **Expression**
- **Tone**
- **Diction**
- **Pace**

Women accurately described the situation 87 per cent of the time. Only men involved in 'artistic' or 'nurturing' occupations, such as teaching or nursing, performed as well (Anderson, 1993).

Certainly by acquiring the skill of reading other people's body language and using our own, we may be able to establish rapport more quickly and effectively with audiences. If we allow our body language to leak messages about some of our inflammatory emotions, for example, disgust, fear or irritation, difficulties will arise.

Recent work in the USA within sports psychology, indicates that it may be possible to teach athletes to perform better by getting them to use confident body language. Presenters could use this principle. Confident body language may give you the extra boost you need.

Exercise

Think back to a time when you were really confident. Perhaps during a presentation or even in a social situation. Let the enthusiasm and energy flood in. Try rehearsing a presentation before and after doing this exercise, to see if it makes any difference.

Where do I stand?

Stand where you are comfortable. Experts describe the 'Power Position' as the most effective position.

However, you will need to decide on a visually accessible place for your notes. If you feel more comfortable behind the lectern, then take no notice of those who wax lyrical about dismantling barriers. If you prefer to move

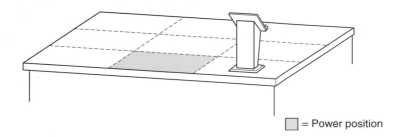

Figure 6.1 Power position.

☐ = Power position

about, that is all right too, as long as your movements are purposeful. For a long time I struggled to control pointless wandering and rocking whilst speaking. I was aware of this distracting habit following feedback from a colleague, which was confirmed once I watched myself on video. Another trainer helped me to correct this bad habit by making me stay in one place for a while, by imagining myself in ski boots, locked to the floor.

Do try to avoid putting your back to a window or a strong light source, as this will tire the audience, make eye contact difficult and offer interesting distractions behind you, not to mention the possibility of your clothes becoming transparent.

How do I stand?

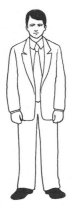

Figure 6.2 The stance to aim for.

Except in unusual circumstances, standing is important whilst giving any presentation. It is tempting to sit, in an attempt to foster an informal atmosphere and to be less conspicuous. However, if you want to produce a change in understanding or opinion, you will need to exert influence. By standing up, you can be more influential and you will be able to move and breathe properly. Do not be tempted to lean on the lectern, as this is sometimes perceived as being too relaxed.

Your feet should be about eight to ten inches apart, with knees slightly bent and not locked. You are then ready to walk in any direction, in a natural and relaxed manner. Put your feet parallel. This may feel funny, but will look fine. Rock slowly and gently back and forth until you can feel that your weight is centred between the front of the arches and the balls of your feet. Once you have established this position, lift your shoulders, but not your arms, and then let your hands fall gently to your sides.

Use your hands to invite the audience to accept your point, by keeping them open with the palms pointing upwards. Leave the front of your body unprotected. If you look defensive, the audience may doubt your credibility and sincerity.

To demonstrate attentiveness you need to lean very slightly forward towards the audience, with uncrossed arms. These principles may seem basic to some of you, but most of us do not stick to them, particularly when under pressure. If you want to see an excellent example of good attending, watch an experienced television presenter. Once they start interviewing a guest, turn the sound down so you cannot hear what they are talking about. Watch how they lean forward and make eye contact. See how they nod their heads. They do not do this mechanically, but they do do it a lot, and you can see the effect it has on their guests. It does not necessarily mean they agree, but it does say 'I'm with you, keep going'. Note how they use their facial muscles. Most of us do not use facial expression very much when we listen to another person. Interviewers are constantly crinkling and furrowing into smiles, and grimacing as their guest sends out a stream of differing emotions (Wylie and Grothe, 1993).

Exercise

Put a mirror next to your phone for a week and watch your face while you are talking. Look for any fake, fierce or gormless expressions you make. Once you are aware of them, you can do something about them. Practice smiling and looking confident.

Experts claim that the best communicators communicate with their whole being. They are animated and exciting to watch. However, many people are too inhibited to be able to use themselves deliberately as a visual aid.

Restrict your movements to those which support your message, to avoid looking as though you are trying to teach the audience to line dance. Presenters are often unaware of their bad habits, such as face touching, scratching or chin rubbing, which can suggest lack of confidence. Experts take the opportunity to review themselves on video frequently. The tape can be fast forwarded to accentuate habitual gestures. Unfortunately, many refuse such opportunities, as they feel too self-conscious. Sadly, they miss the chance to access unfiltered feedback.

Another way to drop bad habits is to write them in large letters on an index card and put them on the lectern during your presentation, as a reminder.

Body language pitfalls

- Swaying from foot to foot
- Jangling jewellery or change in pockets

- Fiddling
- Exaggerated and meaningless gestures
- Moving around and speaking at the same time.

You can use body language to inject the pep-me-ups mentioned in Chapter 2 ('Preparation is the key to success'). To maintain attention you need to change what you have been doing every so often. Perhaps you can do the opposite. If you have been moving around, stop. If you have been standing in one spot, then start to move around.

Exercise

If this is you, try demonstrating appropriate body language to accompany some of the following concepts:

- Nurture creativity
- Manipulate opinion
- Break open a closed mind
- Dodge some of the irrelevant issues
- Face the problem head on
- Confront some of our concerns

as though they were included in your presentation. If gesturing does not come easily to you, force at least one gesture into each sentence during your practice sessions. You will find it starts to come much more naturally.

Eye contact

By keeping your chin up, you will be able to maintain good eye contact with the audience and you will indicate confidence and interest. Humans are the only primate species with visible areas of white framing the iris; this means that even small movements of the eyes are visible from a distance. It is universally accepted that effective eye contact is essential to establish warm, interested relationships. This is another reason to use outline notes rather than a script.

Eye contact needs to be worked at. Studies show that locking eyes with one person in a group has a positive impact on all those present. Poor eye contact can give the impression of anxiety, incompetence, lack of sincerity, lack of credibility and it prevents you from eliciting feedback from the audience.

It is worth remembering that each of us has a bias towards either right or left when looking at a group and we need to consider that bias when getting eye contact right (Van Ments, 1990).

Eye contact pitfalls

- Avoiding sections of the room
- Looking out of the window
- Looking at one spot
- Forgetting the back rows of the audience
- Looking over the heads of the audience.

By making eye contact with individuals, when you mention something relevant to their area of expertise, you will acknowledge their experience. If you concentrate on those looking bored and cynical, and raise your eyebrows occasionally, you will appear friendly and encourage questions. You will also invite the observer to accept your ideas.

Eye contact is very useful when dealing with someone who might be causing trouble in the audience by asking difficult questions. Once they know you are responding with warm, sincere eye contact and treating any concerns as though they are legitimate ones, gently turn your eye contact to others in the audience. Slowly move your eyes away, establishing eye contact with other people as you go, until you are not looking anywhere near the original person. By the time you have finished responding, you are not looking at the difficult person and you will not be giving them visual permission to continue causing trouble.

If you make eye contact with someone who quickly looks away, try not to look directly into that person's eyes again. In some cultures direct eye contact is inappropriate and some individuals just feel uncomfortable being looked at. Any discomfort will get in the way of their concentration.

One cardinal rule when making presentations is: do not talk unless you have eye contact. You may want to start with the people on the front row who are often the most interested and attentive.

Facial expression

As the old Chinese proverb advises 'A man without a smile must not open a shop'. It is difficult for anybody to respond to a smile with anything other than a smile. Even more powerful is a smile starting with the lips and spreading to the eyes. However, smiling inappropriately can create as negative an impression as not smiling at all. A smile plastered on the face of someone who is talking about downsizing their service will only serve to alienate listeners.

Using your voice

The human voice has the power to affect and stimulate emotions in a way that the written word cannot. There is an old saying amongst Members of Parliament that everything depends upon the manner in which one speaks and not upon the matter. Remember that the audience will probably have made up their mind about whether to continue to listen to you within the first couple of minutes of seeing you, and, according to Mehrabian (1972), 38 per cent of your message will be conveyed through your tone of voice. Do not waste this opportunity to create a first impression by asking 'Can you hear me at the back?'. Watch the audience's faces instead.

Before you utter your first words into the microphone, make sure you say a few words to yourself in private, to prevent a squeaky voice. A raised pitch makes the speaker sound unsure or shrill. However, a lowered pitch for an important sentence or at the end of a sentence will add strength and conviction.

Jacobi surveyed a nation-wide sample of 100 men and women and asked 'Which irritating or unpleasant voice annoys you most?'. The answer was a whining, complaining or nagging tone. He claims that people judge our intelligence much more by how we sound than how we dress (Anderson, 1993).

Speakers who have regional accents are sometimes self-conscious, although, as long as they can be understood, they are usually a welcome change. If you speak more slowly and deliberately than usual, the audience should be able to keep up. This sounds rather artificial to your own ears initially, but soon passes. Just imagine speaking to someone for whom English is not the first language. The audience will need at least one minute to adjust to your speech pattern, no matter how clear you are.

Many dialects have natural modulation, for example Irish, where the note in the voice rises and falls. You normally hear your own voice amplified through the bones of your skull, so it sounds different to the voice heard by others. If you do find you have a tendency to be monotonous, it is worth trying the simple media technique of placing stress, inflection or a change of tone on every fifth word or syllable, to give rhythm.

Exercise

Try saying 'forty thousand pounds' quickly and with an air of triviality, so that it sounds like a very small sum. Then try 'four thousand pounds' with feeling. Say it as though you are staggered by the huge amount of money. The four thousand will probably sound huge, whilst the forty thousand will sound like peanuts.

Verbal pitfalls

- Speech slurry. 'Ums' and 'ers' get in the way. Eventually audiences can become so distracted they start to count these useless fillers. You can overcome this bad habit, through feedback, during rehearsal. A trusted colleague or friend can indicate to you when you use speech slurry, by raising a hand, beeping or ringing a bell
- Filler words are a problem. Three favourite fillers are 'generally speaking', 'actual' and 'basically'. You may have other words you slip in when you are not thinking
- Any bad language or discriminatory remarks
- Mispronunciation of words can often cause listeners to consider speakers to be poorly educated and not very clever
- Repetition is the mother of retention. When a point is repeated it suggests to the audience that it is a crucial one. Make sure that any that are repeated are crucial. If you stumble over a word or phrase several times during rehearsal, change it, do not risk it
- Dropping your voice at the end of a sentence. This becomes too difficult to listen to, and content is lost

Repetition is the mother of retention

- Slurred or mumbled words will eventually irritate an audience, as they will have to strain to understand you
- Failure to pause long enough between ideas. Listeners need time to reflect on what they have heard
- Pitching your voice inappropriately.

Exercise

Audio tape yourself reading a children's book aloud for ten minutes. Concentrate on projection, diction and pace. Repeat the exercise three times a week.

Further tips

ALWAYS:
- Be positive and enthusiastic
- Pause between ideas
- Repeat key points
- Pitch your voice appropriately

AVOID:
- Mispronunciation
- Filler words – umm, er, 'generally speaking', 'actual', 'basically'.
- Jokes during the introduction

NEVER:
- Use discriminatory remarks
- Offensive language
- Drop your voice at the end of sentences
- Tell long, involved stories

Periods of silence or prolonged pauses are useful to regain audience attention. Such silences can be as long as five or six seconds, without feeling uncomfortable to the audience. Pace of presentation, that is, how quickly or slowly you speak, makes a difference as well.

If you tend to scatter speech slurry into your presentations or your diction is not as clear as it could be, work on improving it every day. If you can make improvements on daily interactions, it will carry over into the presentation setting.

Passive sentences are power robbers: 'the patient was turned by me' as opposed to 'I turned the patient'. Two of the most powerful words we have are 'You' and 'I' and we do not use them enough in the context of presentations.

Exercise

Stand in a lecture room and imagine that you are throwing a big rubber ball to the corner of the room. As it leaves your hands, call to an imaginary person to catch the ball. Feel the words leaving your mouth and direct them to the person.

Humour

People like laughing. People tend to like people who make them laugh, and if they like you, they will usually listen more carefully to what you say. Using humour in your presentations is not about telling jokes. You do not have to be John Cleese or Rosanne Arquette to use humour effectively during presentations. A positive and enthusiastic approach is much more valuable than being able to tell jokes confidently. Amusing real-life stories can relieve tension, relax and actually help people learn or remember. There are some pitfalls though, which can be avoided.

> Analysing humour is like dissecting a frog. Few people are interested and the frog dies of it
>
> *E.B. White (author of Charlotte's Web)*

Humour pitfalls

- Embarrassing other people
- Using dialects or telling discriminatory jokes
- Spoiling a joke by letting the audience know you are going to tell one
- Using an unconnected joke
- Going overboard on poking fun at yourself
- Putting all your eggs in one basket by using one long joke or funny story. If you use five one-liners rather than one long joke, you have five chances at success.

You may find it helpful to ask yourself the following questions.
Would you tell the joke:

- To your mother or grandmother?
- To a religious leader?
- If it were to be broadcast to the whole country?
- To everyone in the health centre coffee room at lunch time?

Practise by telling your story or joke several times, in the funniest way possible, until you feel comfortable telling it. Try sneaking it into everyday conversations, but do not start with 'do you think this is funny?'.

You have heard jokes that have fallen flat. These failures are accompanied by a painful silence, with everyone feeling uncomfortable. People assume that jokes are ice breakers, but they can break much more than ice. For this reason I avoid jokes during the introduction.

The most natural expression of humour is a simple smile. Do not worry about not deliberately incorporating humour. Most people find something that is naturally funny to laugh at, for example, an upside-down slide or an unfortunate noise. Do not take yourself too seriously and your natural sense of humour will come through. Even the Talmud teaches that a lesson taught with humour is a lesson retained.

> Laughter is no enemy to learning
>
> *Walt Disney*

Timing

Do not look at your watch whilst you are speaking. You may give the message that you have had enough and want to go. During the 1992 election campaign, President Bush was debating with Bill Clinton and Ross Perot, when he took a long look at his watch. Nobody remembers his verbal message that day.

Many dread having to speak after lunch when people are using all of their energy on digestion, which draws energy away from the brain. The other more challenging time is 3–4 p.m., when the liver is often at its lowest ebb. If you can, you may like to avoid these times unless your presentation involves lots of humour, excitement, interaction or movement.

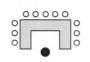

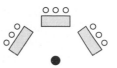

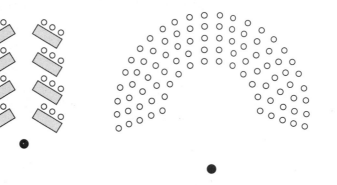

Figure 6.3 Four examples of good seating configurations for presentations.

Setting up the room

There are only three excuses for being late or not turning up at your own presentation: a death in the family, serious illness or critical injury. By arriving at the venue at least one hour before the start of your session, you can sort out almost any problem with the layout. Do not assume that the room will be set up in a way that is most suitable for presentations. One way to avoid difficulties on the day is to get good information from the organizers, and to make sure they are clear about your requirements. I usually put these in writing so there are no misunderstandings.

Once you arrive you should check the 'ATLS':

- Aids
- Temperature
- Lighting
- Seating.

Aids

Trust nobody but yourself to check any equipment you might need. As in clinical practice, it is frightening to turn confidently to a piece of equipment, only to find it is not working. You need to check the sound system and any visual aids (see more about this in Chapter 3). It is well worth learning the names of the technical staff on site who can protect you against audio-visual disaster.

Tip

Find out the names of the technical support staff at the venue.

Temperature

Make sure the temperature of the room is on the cool side. Once it is filled with bodies, a great deal of heat will be generated and warm atmospheres lead quickly to sleepiness. Find out the contact name for the person able to adjust the temperature as soon as you arrive.

Lighting

Natural light is lovely to work in, but windows at a venue can be a nightmare. Audience attention can wander, sun shines in and distracts. If windows are unavoidable, try to make sure the audience has its back to them. The general rule for lighting is to keep it bright for maximum excitement. If the lights do need to be dimmed for a slide presentation, turn them back up as soon as possible.

Seating

Remove any spare chairs, as twenty-five people in a room with fifty chairs makes the venue look empty. Again, you need to check who to contact and how to contact them if there is a problem.

If you set up 30 per cent fewer chairs than the number you will expect, but have extra chairs available, a last minute rush to find seats will add energy and excitement.

Will everyone be able to see? Sit in different parts of the room and check. Will they be comfortable? Up to thirty people can be seated in a semicircle, and up to fifty in a double semicircle. When seats are placed in rows, the audience members are unable to make eye contact with each other, which is important to them so that they can see how others are responding.

If you place seats so that the audience are facing you with their backs to the door, those who are late can slip in. Try to keep a few vacant chairs here so that latecomers will not have to stumble around to find a seat. Use masking tape to cover the metal latches of the doors leading into the room, so that when they close there will be very little sound.

If you are speaking in an auditorium and the seats are all fixed, it is worth taping along the aisles at the back, to stop the audience spreading out from the back and then being asked to move nearer to the front.

Winston Churchill insisted that the rebuilt House of Commons should not have as many seats as there were MPs, in an attempt to make the House feel as full as possible.

It is very important to sort out seating arrangements before the audience arrives. People tend to resent being moved after they have entered a room and sat down.

The distance between the audience and any visual aid screen should be no more than six times the width of the projected image. There must be enough distance between the screen and the first row of chairs: approximately twice the width of the screen. All seating should be within thirty feet of the screen.

When the audience have to keep turning their heads to watch you and to see the slides, they quickly become uncomfortable and therefore less receptive to your message. Test the seating provided for you by sitting in the outermost seats with the equipment turned on.

It is worth sitting in the audience yourself, before your presentation, to check for any problems. It was only by sitting at the back of a lecture hall with time to spare, that I noticed the terrible draught blowing across the room. I also realized how noisy the slide projector was, and could take measures to rectify these problems in time for my presentation. You can also use the opportunity at break time to start mingling with the audience to ask whether there are any difficulties from their point of view. Networking with others will start to generate some support for you before you have even stood up to speak.

Is the route to the podium clear? If you are talking to a small group you should not stand on a higher level. Close any windows overlooking a busy street to avoid distracting noise. Can you see the correct time? If not, either put your watch on the lectern or on the inside of your wrist, so you can take subtle glances at it.

Finally, prepare your glass of water in advance. Fill it only half full and put it somewhere sensible.

Briefing the Chair

Chairing a meeting or conference is a skill in itself. Sadly, not all chairpersons realize this. They wait until a few moments before your presentation to find out your name and sometimes seem to guess the rest. One way to avoid a blundering introduction is to provide the chairperson with written details well in advance. You can write your own introduction, highlighting the relevant areas and why you will be speaking. This should be typed, with double spacing, at least 18 font and it should take less than ninety seconds to read. You can then avoid the chair:

- Giving your main message themselves
- Taking too much of your presentation time
- Boring the audience
- Giving you a build-up you can never live up to.

Sometimes conference organizers are tempted to place the Chair and other speakers at a table on the platform, where they are sure to move occasionally. Each time they make the slightest movement, the audience will be distracted. People cannot resist the temptation to look at anything that moves, so try to make sure that you avoid such distractions if possible.

Resuscitating a flagging audience

Research conducted in the USA looked at a group of students asked to attend a series of lectures. Each student was instructed to keep their legs uncrossed, arms unfolded and to take a casual relaxed sitting position. At the end of the lecture the retention of each student was tested and their attitude toward the lecturer noted. A second group of students was put through the same process, but these students were told to keep their arms tightly folded across their chests throughout the lecture. Results showed that the group with the folded arms retained 38 per cent less than the unfolded arms group. The second group also had a more critical opinion of the lecture and the lecturer. Perhaps this underlines the importance of comfort when listeners are to retain a message.

The average passive adult attention span is about thirteen minutes in the UK, which seems to be reducing year on year. There is a theory that this is the result of television. Other evidence shows that people listen intently for only three seconds out of every ten. You need to search for feedback from the audience constantly to check they are hearing you.

How can you tell?

- Look for facial expressions indicating interest, impatience, distress, enthusiasm, puzzlement, irritation, boredom or acceptance
- Watch the angle at which people's bodies are positioned. Leaning forward indicates interest. Leaning backwards can indicate lack of interest or merely tiredness
- Are their arms or legs crossed or are their hands over their mouths, which may indicate hostility or lack of interest?
- Are they looking around the room for something more interesting?
- Coughing or throat clearing seems to spread as though everyone is waiting for someone else to start
- Nodding is a very reassuring sign.

If you are still not sure, then ask some questions to see whether the audience are alert and understanding you. You have already decided what your 'end' is. Is the audience getting there? If you are starting to lose them, go back. Re-emphasize why they need to listen to you. Remind them of the WAM factor. Make a loud noise as part of the content or do something unusual. Change the style of the session or, even better, stop the audience drifting off in the first place. Remember that just one word out of place can leave the audience behind, puzzling over the meaning. Keep it short and simple (KISS).

If you decide to take a comfort break, you may find it difficult to recapture attention. By blowing softly into the

> The mind can only absorb what the behind can endure
>
> *Mark Twain*

microphone, you should find that chatter soon comes to a halt. Alternatively you can announce 'If you can hear me please clap twice'. Once you have repeated this a few times, you will find your listeners will be applauding and you will be ready to begin.

Once you have completed your presentation, rather than looking down away from the audience, leaving the stage, or gathering your notes, stand in the centre of the stage, look directly at the audience and acknowledge their applause by saying a quiet 'Thank you'.

Summary

Investing the time to prepare your venue, so that it is the best it possibly can be, is well worth the effort. Getting up there in front of the audience is the most difficult part of making a presentation, for me. However, if I keep the focus on the audience, rather than on myself, I can concentrate on the job I have to do rather than on how well I am performing. A starting ritual has been invaluable to help me keep focused and prevent panic. Once you can walk out and speak in front of other people, you can start to concentrate on finer details, like reading body language and using eye contact. There are one or two pitfalls you really must avoid, such as making tasteless jokes or being monotonous. Otherwise, there is a great deal of scope. You can try different approaches and develop your own style.

References

Anderson, K. (1993) *Getting What You Want*. Penguin, London.
Mehrabian, A. (1972) *Non Verbal Communication*. Aldine Atherton, Chicago.
Van Ments, M. (1990) *Active Talk – The Effective Use of Discussion in Learning*. Kogan Page, London.
Wylie, P. and Grothe, M. (1993) *Dealing with Difficult Colleagues*. Piatkus, London.

7 Handling questions

The question and answer section of your presentation may
well be the most important part. It allows the audience to
raise their concerns, it enables you to check their level of
understanding and it allows you to tie up loose ends. Many
new presenters dread questions at the end of their presentation. They recognize that a good presentation with a
poor question and answer session will spoil the overall
effect. Conversely, though, a poor presentation can be
saved by good questions and answers.

The key, as usual, is preparation. You need to spend as
much time rehearsing the answers to questions as you
spend preparing the presentation itself. Then, instead of
dreading questions, you can treat each one as an indication
of interest and respond positively. The cardinal rule for
questions is: do not put them right at the end. It moves the
audience's focus from your message and can introduce
doubts. The best place for questions is just before your
conclusion.

Before your presentation you need to be clear about:

- When to take questions, at the end or during your
  session. Questions taken at any time need a confident
  speaker to control proceedings. However, by leaving
  questions to the end, you may frustrate the audience or
  they may forget their question. A good compromise may
  be to take questions at the end of each section
- How to prompt them. Do you want the chairman to
  manage them or will you do it yourself? You will need to
  encourage questions with positive words and body
  language. 'What questions do you have?' works so
  much better than 'Any questions?'. The first is an open

question but the second is a closed one, crying out for the answer, 'No'. By raising your hand when you ask 'Who has a question?' You can take advantage of the 'mirroring principle'. If you put your hand up, members of the audience are much more likely to raise theirs. Wait at least five seconds with a friendly look on your face
- How you plan to answer them. It is fairly easy to anticipate questions you are likely to be asked. By putting these on separate pieces of paper or index cards, you can formulate the answers in anticipation
- Whether anything in your presentation is contentious
- Whether people want to know more about anything
- Whether you have made any claims which may need further proof
- Whether anyone has an axe to grind.

Tips
Questions and Answers should:

- Emphasise key messages
- Be controlled by the speaker
- Involve the audience

Have you ever wondered how the Prime Minister can answer questions posed at press conferences so well? He may not know exactly what Tom, Dick or Harriet are going to ask him, but he does know what is likely to come up, and he prepares for it.

One colleague asks listeners to fill out blank index cards with questions, before the presentation begins. She then refers to them throughout her presentation. However, she also has her own cards on which questions she can, and wishes to, answer are written. By using this trick, she emphasizes her key messages, retains control and involves the audience.

Tips for handling questions

- Anticipate everything and leave nothing to chance. Practise your presentation in front of others and encourage them to ask difficult questions
- If you are taking questions throughout, it is fine to ask questioners to wait a moment whilst you finish making a

point. However, always come back to them if you say you will

- By moving around the audience during question time, you can encourage participation
- Listen carefully right to the end of the question. By listening to the first few words, some presenters try to guess the rest of the question, and then answer incorrectly or inappropriately
- Take your time to respond, do not react. Make sure you are quite clear of the question before you try to answer it
- Ensure the question is heard and understood by the audience, by repeating it. You can also use this time to formulate your answer
- Stepping towards your questioner shows you are prepared and confident
- Try to avoid the tendency to say 'That's a good question' before you answer it
- When answering, adhere to KISS principles (Keep It Short and Simple). Answer in one sentence, followed by a supporting statement or example and link it in with your presentation somewhere
- Give the questioner two-thirds of your eye contact whilst delivering the answer. The other third can cover the rest of the audience, who will then not feel comfortable to whisper to the person next to them
- Always, always respond positively, no matter how hostile or stupid the question seems
- Do not be defensive
- Avoid being untruthful
- Never repeat someone's negative point of view in your answer to a question. For example 'Why have you allowed such ridiculously long delays for patients between them sustaining their fractured neck of femur and surgery?'
- Do not return to the person who asked the question and ask them if you have answered it. If you need to ask, you probably have not but the rest of the audience probably do not care, so avoid a detailed discussion with one person and keep it moving. If facial expression and body language suggest a problem, seek out the questioner at the end of the session to sort out any difficulties which remain
- If someone asks a question that will be covered later on, say so. Avoid lengthy responses which will interrupt your train of thought and lose the audience's interest.

> ## Further tips
>
> ALWAYS be positive
> NEVER be defensive or untruthful.

You must behave as if you cannot wait for the questions. If you timidly ask ' Are there any questions?', that begs the answer 'No'. You need to step forward and ask 'What questions can I answer for you?'. Pause for a few seconds and raise your hand if you would like them to do so. Alternatively, you could ask 'Is everyone happy with that?', 'What problems do you see?', or 'What uncertainties remain?'.

Patrick Collins (1998) suggests that when you conduct a question and answer session, you think R.E.S.T. – that is:

- **R**espond
- **E**xample – give one
- **S**top talking
- **T**ake next question.

This will allow you to organize your thoughts better, focus on ideas and issues and keep your answers to about the same length.

Handling difficult situations

Controversial areas

Try to find some common ground at the beginning of your presentation. If you start with the least controversial issues, you can get agreement and then move on to the more difficult areas. You can remind the audience of your common ground if the situation gets rocky and, once again, when calling for action at the end.

You do not know the answer

Do not be afraid to say you do not know, but always say you will try to find out, and then do so: 'I don't know the answer, but, if you leave your contact details, I'll phone or fax you tomorrow'. Another tactic involves redirecting the question to the questioner or to the audience: 'How would some of you deal with that?'.

Several questions in one

Ask for the main question and answer that, or pick one part for yourself and answer it. Also, you could acknowledge the questions, ask that the questioner write them down and offer to answer them after the presentation.

No questions

To avoid an uncomfortable silence, you could ask for written questions in advance of your presentation, or plant a questioner in the audience to avoid this situation. However, if it does happen, you can break the ice by saying 'all right, we'll start with the *second* question'. You can ask if anyone would like to comment on your presentation, but do not allow any sublectures. Ask the audience a question. Alternatively, you could say you were asked a question privately, or 'I'm often asked' or 'What do you think about?'.

Once you have answered your own question say 'Now, what other questions can I answer?'. This usually works. If all else fails offer to take questions privately.

Handling difficult questioners

No matter what kind of problem these questioners are, avoid embarrassing them at all costs. It is essential to remain positive at all times. Once you respond sarcastically or negatively to anyone in the audience, their fellow listeners will react to protect them and you will find yourself faced with a hostile audience. You are in a powerful position and audiences object to seeing that power abused, no matter how badly the questioner is behaving.

Hostile

Often these people have a hidden agenda. You can expose this by asking 'Do you have some thoughts on ... ?'. Very occasionally, individuals will make openly hostile comments. By saying 'That's an interesting point, let's see what the rest of the audience think of it', you can let the audience handle this aggression themselves whilst you remain positive. 'That's not a position we've looked at before. Perhaps we can explore it at the next session' can also work well.

Keep on trying to find some common ground. Minimize the differences and keep drawing them back to the point being made. Do not answer a negatively loaded question until you change it to a neutral one: for example, 'How come your waiting lists for surgery are so horrendously long?' to 'Let me identify some of the delays experienced by some of our patients waiting for surgery'.

Mini lecturer

Do not allow anyone to dominate, either with lots of questions or by lengthy responses. If someone is rambling, wait for a pause, thank them and then restate the relevant point they have made. You could also politely interrupt and say 'Let me see if I understand your comment/question'. Summarize the speaker's words and then respond appropriately. You can ask listeners to put their questions in writing and pass them to the front. This helps them put together more concise questions and allows you to rephrase them if necessary.

Show off

Avoid embarrassing these individuals. Ask yourself 'Why are they behaving this way?'. Usually they need to feel heard for some reason. Let them have a little of the limelight and then use the 'See you at Coffee' technique. You can express great interest in what they have to say and explain that time is short so you would like to meet at coffee to discuss the issue further. You have acknowledged how interesting and clever they are, and limited the mini lecturer potential.

Digresser

Sometimes a member of the audience misses the point completely and starts to digress. You can avoid embarrassment by taking the blame yourself. 'I must have led you away from the main issue. Remember we are discussing ...'. Otherwise you can say 'Certainly that's something I need to clarify. Perhaps I can pick it up in context.'

Whisperers

Avoid embarrassing them. Address a point to them by name if you can or repeat the last point and ask for comments.

Confused or inarticulate

Respond with 'Let me repeat that' and do it in a clearer way. If the question is really off beam you could say 'That's one way of looking at it, but how do we reconcile that with (correct point)'.

Summary

Always make sure you end your question and answer section on a strong note. If you ask for 'One more question, please', you may take an irrelevant or hostile one which will create an ending to your presentation like a damp squib. I would recommend you cover questions before taking two to three minutes to draw conclusions. That way, no new information is introduced after the presentation is complete.

If you can end your question and answer session before the audience runs out of questions, you can keep energy high for the closure. You may want to say 'We've almost run out of time. I will be happy to stay around to answer any remaining questions, or you can phone me.'

After you answer the last question, restate your main points and then leave them with the 'end'. What do you want them to do now?

Reference

Collins, P.J. (1998) *Say it with Power and Confidence*. Prentice-Hall Direct, Vermont.

8 Dealing with difficult people

Many 'would-be' presenters dread the prospect of a difficult audience. In reality, of course, the vast majority of audiences want you to be a success, they want to learn from you. However, there may be times when others disagree with the message we are presenting. Whenever people disagree about something, the tendency is not to try to see things from the other person's point of view. The natural tendency is to assume that the other person does not know what they are talking about. When handling difficult situations we need to minimize potential damage. As with many issues in life, it is not what happens, it is how you handle it.

Studies consistently show that, in most situations, people respond better to praise of their positive behaviours, rather than to punishment for their negative ones. For example, if I wanted to make sure you always considered pain control as a priority for patients in sickle cell crisis, I would have more success if I praised you when you made analgesia a priority than if I moaned at you when you did not.

When dealing with difficult participants, your goals are:

1 to get the difficult person on board
2 to minimize negative impact on any other participants.

Tips for dealing with difficult people

- Always face a difficult situation straight away
- Never embarrass anyone in front of a group
- Never show you are angry during a presentation
- Concentrate on the audience not yourself.

Occasionally you may be faced with a difficult audience. Sometimes they appear uninformed and apathetic. For these groups it is essential to grab their attention early on. Information needs to be carefully explained, given a little at a time, repeated with variations and with plenty of examples. Stress your own expertise and use lots of successful role models and examples. Usually, though, you will only have to cope with difficult individuals.

As for the individuals who may give cause for concern, adhere to the principles above and we will explore different ways of handling them.

Lesley Latecomer

Take particular care when someone arrives into the presentation late. Do not draw attention to them and avoid recapping for their benefit, unless they are the key person for whom the session has been set up. If the room has several doors, make sure all except the one you want latecomers to enter through are locked as your session starts. Try rewarding those who arrive on time with praise.

Preoccupied Pat

These individuals write notes, arrange their papers and read during your session. One way to control this is to make sure that the organizers provide personal storage areas. That way, audience members are separated from some of the things they are preoccupied with.

Hassling Hilary

Hassling Hilary's aim seems to be to interrupt and cause trouble. He usually has a specific point he wants to make, and he makes that point in ways that interrupt the flow of your presentation, prevent others from asking questions and intimidate you.

These individuals can add energy if you use them. Do not fight fire with fire, though. Stay warm and positive at all costs and act as though they are being curious and helpful. If you act as though each member of the audience will behave with honour and consideration, you will at least get better behaviour. As soon as possible, involve them in a task that requires follow up, for example, keeping the presenter to time or capturing ideas on the flip chart.

If they have already started causing trouble, look them straight in the eye and listen to what they have to say. Pause for a few seconds to think about what they are challenging, looking as comfortable as possible. Respond with a sincere answer.

Talkative Tony

These people talk non-stop to anyone who will listen, including you. They will offer an opinion on everything. To interrupt the talk-hog, lean towards them, point your finger in the air, wait for them to take a breath and quickly interject with 'Let me respond to that' then respond and turn away. Do not make eye contact again and move the focus. 'We've not heard from the back/front/left/right', in fact anywhere other than where the talk-hog is.

Chin-wagger Charlie

The Talkative Tony who has no joy with you, will try to talk to everyone else. You can try simply lowering your voice, making Charlie's conversation louder in contrast, often resulting in other people asking them to be quiet. You can also smile warmly in their direction and say 'Good, a question ... Oh sorry, I thought you were raising your hand'. By focusing your eyes and voice on Charlie, you can indicate that they are causing a distraction, but on no account embarrass them.

Moaning Max

Moaning Max complains frequently and focuses on the negative. They seem to express dissatisfaction with everything. This attitude spreads like wildfire. Look for some common ground with them and what they are saying. If you can get this individual to share some responsibility for the success of the presentation, they can be very supportive. These individuals will often complain about things over which they have little control, for example, funding of the health service. Gently remind them that the group is unable to influence government policy, but you can explore ways of making better use of resources.

Timid Terry

Timid Terrys stand back and do not participate. Do not focus on these people too early, or you will frighten them off. Give them a chance to see you in action and to see that you will not make a fool of them or put anyone on the spot. In smaller groups, by encouraging short, small buzz groups, you can often break the ice. Ask these people easy questions to get them involved, such as 'Is the room too hot or too cold?'.

Know-it-all Nicky

Nickys tell everyone how important they are and have the final word on everything. Beware of embarrassing these individuals. Make sure you acknowledge their status and ask them to share their opinions and experience. If you can identify these individuals before your presentation, you could enlist their help before they can become a problem. You could ask for their opinion or for feedback once your presentation is complete. This is where your contact at the venue is essential. When fully briefed, you can be privy to the most valuable information.

Summary

Remember, nobody wants to see you fail. There will be far more people in the audience who want to learn from you than there are occasional difficult people. Even though there may be members of the audience who are experts in your field, they are NOT expert in what you are going to talk about. I frequently attend presentations on the art of making presentations and I have yet to come away from one having learned nothing at all. I always hear a new tip or a colourful story. I also listen to new ways of explaining difficult areas, which I can use later with participants at my own seminars.

On the rare occasion when you do meet with someone difficult or hostile in your audience, when you handle them well you can generate extra credibility. However, no matter how skilled or knowledgeable you are, if you manage the situation badly, your reputation will suffer. Above all else, do as much as you can to avoid embarrassing anyone.

9 Proactive media relations

'My name is Laura Humphries and I'm the Health Correspondent with the *Independent*. We want to do a piece on nurses and their changing role in primary care. Are you interested in working with me?'

What would your reaction be? Probably to get away as soon as possible. There is a strong feeling among health care professionals that you cannot trust journalists and they will trick you into making a fool of yourself or misrepresent you in some way. Rather than call this chapter 'Managing the media', I renamed it 'Proactive media relations'; this reflects some interesting experiences I have had when involved with newsworthy items.

A decade ago, my reaction to media coverage was always defensive. When faced with reporters in an Accident & Emergency Department following the fire at Kings Cross in 1987, I gave bland information such as 'The staff have responded very well and all concerned are as well as can be expected'. I was then surprised when journalists disguised themselves as injured patients, infiltrated the hospital and reported sensitive information without consent from patients or staff.

Following a serious rail crash at Cannon Street in London, media issues were handled in a different manner. Experts from the Regional Health Authority were involved early on in the proceedings and press worked alongside paramedics, police, nurses, doctors and administrators to report events as accurately and as quickly as possible. The results were startlingly different. Patients cooperated in news bulletins, it was possible to appeal for people and information and everyone involved felt they had been able to do their job properly. By building strong relations with the media, we can access large audiences when it is necessary to pass important messages to large numbers of people.

Principles of proactive media relations

1 Be open and honest. Plainly, confidentiality may be an issue, but if you are able to speak from the heart, with no bluffing, you will build on strong foundations.
2 Do not let your mouth run away with you. During a presentation at an international conference, I made a few rather amusing comments about a medical colleague. These were both unnecessary and unkind. Although I had asked that any members of the press should leave the conference hall before I started my presentation, one reporter stayed and my insulting comments were turned into headlines when the evening paper appeared. I hurt a colleague, reflected badly on my trust and showed myself up as lacking in honour, all for indulging in an entertaining throw-away line. Think about the impact of every word before you speak it.
3 Use the public relations officer linked with your organization. Most trusts have an identified individual who handles contact with the media. Make sure you keep them fully informed if you are involved in any publicity. They often have strong links with individuals and can provide invaluable advice.
4 Prepare, prepare, prepare. Make sure you do all your homework before any interview. I find it helps to practise key phrases beforehand. You can anticipate many of the questions you will be asked and can practise answering them.
5 Court the media. Keep in touch with any journalist or presenter with whom you have worked in the past. There will often be times in the future when you can help each other. I worked with a local journalist on a number of occasions. We had met when winter bed crises were hitting our hospital and a number of unfavourable reports had appeared in the local press. We talked on the telephone and agreed a strategy that we would talk every two weeks and discuss any important issues which might interest readers. Some weeks we reported on what measures were being taken to alleviate waits in the

Accident and Emergency Department, at others we ran features on trauma training for doctors and nurses and once we wrote about our problems with theft of crutches, wheelchairs and pillows from the hospital. We even had some of that equipment returned as a result.

6 Seek training. If you will be using the media frequently to reach large audiences, it is well worth seeking media training. A number of organizations provide such training, many of which can be contacted via your public relations representative.

Futher tips

Key principles:
- Be open and honest BUT watch what you say
- Use the professionals if available
- Court the media

But above all:
- Prepare, prepare, prepare
- Seek training

What shall I do if I am approached?

1 Find out their angle. This simply means you need to find out why it is that what you have to say may be newsworthy.

2 Why have they approached you? Is there someone who may be better informed or more experienced at dealing with the media? Have they already approached anyone else?

3 Identify the journalist and their paper or station. If it is a radio or television programme, is it to be recorded or broadcast live? There are risks associated with being recorded. If the interview is edited, you can end up appearing to support a message you did not intend (Urech, 1997).

4 If you are approached by telephone, make sure you write all the details down.

5 What is their deadline? Do not be pushed. Always say you will get back to them. You need time to mull over information and to discuss it with colleagues.

Do your homework

Link key phrases to key points

Make sure you have carefully researched the area on which you will be questioned. I once appeared on one of the popular daytime chat shows and did a whole weekend of research. When the programme was shown on television, I spoke for no more than thirty-five seconds and had time to make one point only. Nevertheless, I was fully prepared, which gave me a great deal of confidence. You will need some facts to convince the audience you are credible; however, overdoing statistics and numbers will destine your contribution to the cutting room floor.

To be prepared, no matter how long your contribution is likely to be, as for a presentation you need to pick your three to five main points. Matched to each of the three to five main points should be a key phrase. You will then have a better chance of making short, succinct points which are included in the programme, rather than rambling, dithery monologues which are eventually cut.

To avoid some of the more vitriolic criticism, it is worth taking a balanced view of your subject. It is important to plan what you want to say, as well as what you do not want to say. You can rest assured that if there is a sensitive area you would rather avoid, any good journalist will ask you questions about it. How will you respond without losing your dignity or credibility?

Who will your audience be? Find out by watching or listening to the programme or reading the paper. There are different audiences for the *Sunday Telegraph* and *TFI Friday*, and your approach will need to reflect this. I watched a Professor of Surgery on the *Big Breakfast* one morning responding to the presenter's questions as though he were addressing gastrointestinal surgeons, not teenagers. His message was both interesting and important, but couched in such specialist terms that only specialists would have understood it.

Know your audience and pitch the level accordingly

As is the case for standard presentations, colourful examples and anecdotes keep your audience interested.

Tips for interviews

1 No notes. Notes during presentations are fine. However, when you appear on television or radio you will not be allowed to take notes in with you, as they can distract

the audience. Under these circumstances, preparation becomes even more vital.

2 Never say anything off the top of your head. As a student nurse, I once commented on the death of a famous patient by telephone to someone I assumed was a friend. My comments appeared in a tabloid newspaper the next day, breaching confidentiality in a most fundamental way.

3 Beware of commenting 'off the record'. Not everyone is honourable. Wait until you have built a strong relationship with journalist colleagues before trusting them with your reputation.

4 Human interest enlivens. Whatever your focus, by weaving in human interest you will make sure your message is received.

5 Avoid jargon. This is even more important with general audiences. Any specialist terms will exclude members of your audience and they will lose your message.

6 Respond carefully to silences. There can be a great temptation to fill silences during an interview. Presenters and journalists will sometimes use them to encourage you to say more than you had planned. Do not say anything you had not planned to say.

Radio

Usually when health care professionals feature on the radio, they have two to three minutes at the most to make their point. On the radio you will be relying solely on how your voice sounds, your appearance will count for nothing (Stuttard, 1997). Does your voice reflect the kind of impression you want to make? Remember that the microphone will be very sensitive. Sometimes radio interviewers will conduct interviews by telephone. If you are expecting such a call, do make sure that:

- You are ready
- You have prepared your key phrases
- You are in a quiet place where you will not be interrupted.

Television

Television audiences are used to short, sharp bursts of information. It is essential to prepare properly for such interviews. Once in the hot seat, put your hands in your lap and your bottom right back on the chair. Keep your head still and slightly nearer to the presenter than you would have it when talking with a friend. Do not look into the camera unless you are told to. Be careful of your facial expression when you are introduced, as it can easily look smug, this is particularly important when being interviewed about a serious subject. I spoiled an opportunity when being interviewed about the effects of Post Traumatic Stress Disorder by keeping an inane grin on my face whilst talking about the suffering of others. Finally, you do not need to thank the interviewer at the end of the interview.

Newspapers

> Reporters are like alligators. You don't have to love them, you don't necessarily have to like them, but you do need to feed them.
>
> *Bowman (1998)*

Journalists will often ask open questions to elicit opinions. Do not try to avoid answering if you are not sure of your reply. Simply say that you do not have all the facts, that you are awaiting a report or that you are unable to reply and why. Do not wait for the journalist to ask you the right question. If you have a pressing message to pass on, make sure it is raised early. Be sure to correct any inaccuracies politely but firmly. Those looking after patients tend to be good at dealing with people, so try if you can to meet with the journalist face to face. Also, you will feel more comfortable on your own territory so try to get them to come to you.

> **Do not say more than you intended: beware of filling silence.**

What to wear for television

Pale grey suits and pale blue shirts work very well. Narrow stripes, checks or hound's-tooth checks can have a strobe effect on a television screen and bright reds can bleed (Stuart, 1996). Avoid large patterns and shiny jewelry which may distract your audience. Women should wear an outfit which buttons down the front, so that a microphone can be attached. Silk often rustles and should be avoided.

   Women should consider wearing heavier make-up than they would usually. Television lighting is so strong it can easily bleach out colouring. It can also get very hot under the studio lights, causing perspiration. Audiences may interpret this as you being uncomfortable with what you are saying. Lots of powder can help both men and women to avoid a shiny face or head.

Before agreeing, ask yourself:

1 What is in it for you or the patient? If there is nothing, why bother?
2 What will benefit your organization and colleagues most?
3 Are you the best person to do this?
4 Is there time to prepare?
5 Do you trust the journalist?
6 What will happen if you refuse?
7 What questions will be asked?

Summary

Once you have asked yourself all these questions, find a colleague to discuss them with. There can be much to be gained for yourself, your colleagues and your patients. However, there is a price to pay if you do not prepare properly. Practising proactive media relations is using a set of skills. Just as you can learn to give a presentation, you can learn these skills also. Many of the skills you have learned to make a presentation also apply to press interviews, but a few other issues must be considered carefully to make sure you reap the great benefits of reaching this wider audience. As well as being able to respond readily to invitations to broadcast, you can seek opportunities to access large audiences.

References

Bowman, D.P. (1998) *Presentations*. Adams Media Corporation, Holbrook, Ma.
Stuart, C. (1996) *How to be an Effective Speaker*. NTC Publishing, Chicago.
Stuttard, M. (1997) *The Power of Public Speaking*. Barrons Educational Series, New York.
Urech, E. (1997) *Speaking Globally*. Kogan Page, London.

10 Publish or perish

Printing was invented in the fifteenth century, heralding a radical change in the way people communicated. It is easy to see the advantages of the written word:

1 People could amend their thoughts before revealing them
2 They could be used as references
3 People in remote places could be communicated with and at unusual times
4 A permanent record could be kept.

The written word helps the reader to understand the author's thoughts, even if the author is not there. The reader can go at his or her own pace and jump forward or backward at will. Sections can be re-read or other written material can be referred to for clarification.

Once you have prepared for a presentation, it is a waste to file all your research, having shared it with only those who were present to hear you speak. You can reach a far wider audience by doing a little more work and having an article published. Many will fall at the first hurdle, not wishing to invest any more time. Others are afraid to commit their ideas to paper. Writing is a durable way of communicating ideas, which makes it a powerful method of reaching many. However, when we write there is always the chance that a colleague will take issue with what we have written. Nevertheless, healthcare professionals are now much better at giving constructive feedback. At least if someone disagrees with what we have written rather than what we have said they will not do it in our presence. Professionals allied to medicine talk so much of wanting recognition for their contributions to patient care, and yet seem unwilling to take the steps required to be recognized. How can any of us be recognized if we do not write or speak formally about what we do?

Twenty years ago standard clinical texts were often written by doctors. At the start of my student nurse training, we were encouraged to purchase *Toohey's Medicine for Nurses* (Bloom, 1978), which was written and edited by a physician. In more recent years the nursing profession has been accused of allowing nurse academics to have too much influence over its development, as journals and book shelves seemed to be filled with the products of academic minds, rather than books and articles aimed at clinical nurses and patient care.

What to write about

Everyone wants to read 'How to . . .' stories: ideas nobody else has had; solutions nobody else has applied; a fresh perspective on an old problem; or a new problem which has not been recognized. You will have covered so many of these areas when preparing for a presentation. It would take me approximately twelve hours to turn a presentation into an article or chapter now, although I am learning to do it more and more quickly. I have found that the more I write, the more confident and competent I become. This is, in part, the result of constant feedback from editors and reviewers.

If you are unsure about whether or not to spend your precious time writing up your presentation, why not contact the editor of a journal or two, outlining who you are and what you are thinking of writing about? You can then ask for details about length of article and authors' guidelines. You should get an idea of how receptive the editor would be to publishing a paper in your area. Remember that one of the most frequent causes of article rejection is that the subject matter is stale. As a general rule, if the subject matter is discussed in general text books, it is already out of date.

Which journal to target

When considering which journal to approach, it is best to familiarize yourself with the style of a few. This means reading approximately four issues from cover to cover, and perusing the section giving advice to authors. Although it is fine to send query letters to a few journals, your finished article should be *submitted to only one.* You may feel your style fits in best with a popular weekly magazine such as *The Health Service Journal*, which has a light journalistic style and articles of 750–2000 words. Some of the heavier monthly journals require academic prose and longer articles, e.g. *International Journal of Nursing Studies*.

Turning your presentation into an article

A good style must first of all be clear

Aristotle

'Start with the end'
Write *something* down on paper.

You already have much of the information you need, it is often simply a matter of breaking the spell and getting started. 'Begin with the end in mind' again. What is the main message you want to convey? Write it on a piece of paper and stick it to your desk, dining room table or computer. Put your reader into your mind's eye and start writing. At first, write anything down. Use a word processor so you will not become too attached to the words; once you have written in long hand, there is a certain reluctance to delete what has taken you some time to commit to paper. If you cannot use a word processor, you need to learn. It is not easy at first, but it is a skill you will require more and more, and it will make life much easier in the long run.

What feedback did you get from your presentation? Reflecting on feedback will help you to decide which areas need emphasis. If you ask for feedback from those present, you should find out which points need further clarification and which could be left out completely.

You will already have three to five main points and will have worked out the flow. Try to limit yourself to one major point every 300 words. Once you have committed something to paper using reasonably short sentences and paragraphs, you should leave it alone for a few days. Try to redo it from memory and then refine and glue it together. By trying to redo from memory, you often come up with clearer ways of explaining difficult areas.

You have already given your message in the spoken word and there is often a temptation to use a completely different set of words and constructions in writing. Do not be tempted. New writers seem addicted to using the passive voice: they write 'It was decided that the patient required physiotherapy three times a day' rather than 'We planned physiotherapy three times a day for the patient'. In the first example who decided? Which sentence is shorter? Research papers are filled with 'It was discovered that' and 'It was observed that'. Does this give the written piece a sense of dignity and objectivity or is it an attempt to make us appear important? Also, why do we keep using long words when short ones will do? The ultimate test of good writing is that it is read and understood by the chosen audience (Albert, 1992).

> **Use active voice rather than passive.**

What if it is rejected?

The most common reasons for rejection are:

1 A boring title. This will be the first, and sometimes the last, opportunity you have to grab your reader's attention. If the title is uninspiring, you will need a committed reader to continue.
2 Failure to hook in the first paragraph. Remember how important first impressions are when making a presentation. A parallel can be drawn with your first paragraph. If you fail to make an impression in the first paragraph or if the content is dull, the reader will not read on.
3 Other people's ideas. If your article is made up of other people's ideas with no conclusions drawn by you, why should people read your piece?
4 A compendium. When writers try to include all they know about a subject, they will end up with a piece which would be more suitable for the *Encyclopaedia Britannica*. If it is too short or too long, your article will be rejected. Stick to the rules.
5 Poor grammar, syntax and spelling. If your article is too difficult to read because it has not been constructed properly or if the spelling is poor, reviewers and editors will not bother to spend the time reading it. If spelling and grammar are not your forte, then pass your article to someone who has skills in this area. When I first started writing, I passed my articles to a law student friend of mine who was very good at making himself clear in writing. Even well-established authors sometimes pass

Most common causes of rejection:

- Boring title
- Weak first paragraph
- Lack of originality
- Too much information
- Poor grammar, syntax and spelling
- Inappropriate focus.

their writing to as many as three people to check for clarity and accuracy.

6 Inappropriate focus. For example, medical not nursing focus for nursing articles. Perhaps nurses are a little sensitive to this issue as a profession. We are seeing many more articles written by nurses in medical journals, and it would be useful to have a balanced approach in nursing journals. Nevertheless, nurses want to read about nursing issues raised by nurses, which is what nursing journal editors will look for.

Summary

Once you have given a presentation, much of the effort required for publication is already done. It is worth putting in that bit of extra time to reach a far wider audience and just for the sheer pleasure of seeing your name in print.

> *If you would not be forgotten*
> *As soon as you are dead and rotten*
> *Either write things worth reading*
> *Or do things worth writing.*
>
> Benjamin Franklin, 1738

References

Albert, T. (1992) *Medical Journalism: The Writers Guide*. Radcliffe Medical Press, Oxford.

Bloom, A. ed. (1978) *Toohey's Medicine for Nurses*, 12th edition. Churchill Livingstone, Edinburgh.

11 Conclusion

Making excellent presentations is a learned skill. Winston Churchill and Abraham Lincoln were both poor speakers in their youth, we are told. They acquired the skill, and you can too, with some preparation and willingness to take a few risks. I have outlined the tips I have accumulated over the last fifteen years of presenting. Sometimes I have performed really well, other times I have embarrassed myself and those present. However, I have kept going. It is rare, now, that I do not deliver effectively. That is a culmination of experience, constant feedback, commitment to improvement and preparation.

However, it matters not whether I have performed well or not. I want people to hear what I say and then to DO something. Perhaps the most rewarding result of giving a successful presentation is to watch the faces of your audience. You can see interest, motivation and admiration. With the progress of advanced communication technology, some assume that traditional presentations will become null and void. However, there is no evidence to support this.

You can improve your performance by reading good literature, using a dictionary and thesaurus and watching able presenters, both amateur and professional. An important part of progressing is to evaluate your own presentation and to ask for feedback. What went well and what could have gone better? If you are really committed to acquiring excellent skills, then seek training. The most valuable part of acquiring training seems to be an increase in confidence.

By finding a mentor and being a mentor you will make faster progress. By being a learner and a teacher at the same time, you will learn faster. However, you must remember that we learn everything by means of gradual improvement. We progress in fits and starts, and often stay still for a while or even slide backwards. Do not get discouraged on the plateaux and abandon your efforts.

You may consider joining one of the Toastmaster groups which are proliferating across this country and elsewhere. These are mixed groups which provide a non-threatening opportunity to gain experience of making presentations, with feedback from others. Initial enquiries should be sent to:

Toastmasters International
PO Box 9052
Mission Viejo
CA 92690
USA

Tel. 714 858 8255
Fax 714 858 1207

> To learn to play the flute, you have to play the flute
>
> *Aristotle*

The most important element of reading this book, as I explained at the beginning, is to close it and then go to prepare a presentation. Whether it is your first or one hundred and first, start afresh with new ideas and a different approach. Once you have presented that one, start on another. When someone asks you to make a presentation say 'Yes, I'll do it', not 'OK, I'll try'.

Use your nerves. Adrenaline heightens your senses, makes you crisper and keeps you alert. But, making presentations is not about your performance. The most important result is that the audience walks away with a message.

What matters is whether you communicate your message to an audience which produces a desired change in understanding or opinion. It is nice to look and sound wonderful too, but the greatest compliment must be 'I see exactly what you mean, I want to go back to my own area now, and do it too'. A test for success is this: someone who was not at your presentation could phone someone who was there, and find out what your message was.

> **Test for success: Have you got your message across – can it be passed on to colleagues who weren't there?**

The difference between a novice and an expert is often only noticeable when something unexpected happens or they make a mistake. The novice makes sure everyone knows about it, through their words, body language and

All the world is on the tip of the tongue

Old Yiddish Proverb

facial expression. The expert knows that it is not what happens but how you handle it. Their verbal and non-verbal cues remain appropriate for the message and they take whatever happens in their stride.

Be yourself, but be your best possible self. Speak about what you believe in and speak from the heart.

Now put the principles into practice!

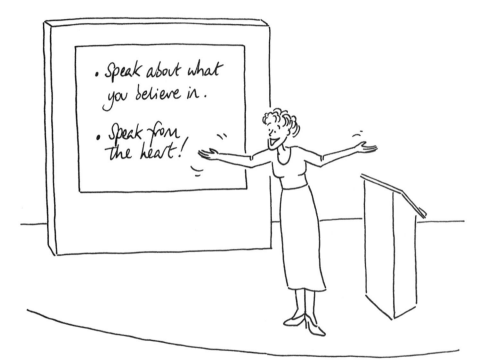

For information about presentation skills seminars and coaching you can contact the author at lisahlaw@aol.com or tel. 01608 811866/fax 01608 811883.

Bibliography

Albert, T. (1992) *Medical Journalism: The Writers Guide*. Radcliffe Medical Press, Oxford.

Anderson, K. (1993) *Getting What You Want*. Penguin, London.

Ashworth, P. (1998) Nurses now read more; what about writing too? *Intensive and Critical Care Nursing*, 14: 107.

Axtell, R.E. (1992) *Do's and Taboos of Public Speaking*. John Wiley & Sons, New York.

Ayres, J. (1988) Coping with speech anxiety: the power of positive thinking. *Communication Education*, 37: 289–296.

Barnum, B.S. (1995) *Writing and Getting Published*. Springer, New York.

Beatty, M.J., Balfantz, G.L. and Kuwabara, A.Y. (1989) Trait-like qualities of selected variables assumed to be transient causes of performance state anxiety. *Communication Education*, 38: 277–289.

Bloom, A. ed. (1978) *Toohey's Medicine for Nurses*, 12th edition. Churchill Livingstone, Edinburgh.

Bowman, D.P. (1998) *Presentations*. Adams Media Corporation, Holbrook, Ma.

Brody, M. (1998) *Speaking Your Way to the Top*. Allyn and Bacon, Needham Heights, Ma.

Brody, M. and Kent, S. (1993) *Power Presentations*. John Wiley & Sons, New York.

Carnegie, D. (1956) *How to Develop Self Confidence and Influence by Public Speaking*. Pocket Books, New York.

Carnegie, D. (1962) *The Quick and Easy Way to Effective Speaking*. Pocket Books, New York.

Collins, P.J. (1998) *Say it with Power and Confidence*. Prentice-Hall Direct, Vermont.

Covey, S.R. (1989) *The Seven Habits of Highly Effective People*. Simon & Schuster, London.

Davies, P. (1990) *Your Total Image*. Piatkus, London.

Desberg, P. (1996) *No More Butterflies*. New Harbinger Publications, Oakland, Ca.

Drott, C., Claes, G., Olsson-Rex, L. *et al*. (1988) Successful treatment of facial blushing by endoscopic transthoracic sympathicotomy. *British Journal of Dermatology*, 138 (4): 639–643.

DuBrin, A.J. (1997) *Personal Magnetism*. AMACOM, New York.

Egan, M. (1998) *Would you Really Rather Die than Talk?* AMACOM, New York.

Gilchrist, D. and Davies, R. (1996) *Winning Presentations*. Gower, London.

Greenberg, D. (1997) *Simply Speaking*. Gold Leaf Publications, Atlanta.

Hasbani, G. (1996) *Winning Presentations*. How to Books, Plymouth.

Hoff, R. (1992) *I Can See You Naked*. Andrews & McMeel, Kansas City.

Hoff, R. (1996) *Say it in Six*. Andrews & McMeel, Kansas City.

Hoff, R. (1997) *Do Not Go Naked into Your Next Presentation*. Andrews & McMeel, Kansas City.

Holcombe, M.W. and Stein, J.K. (1997) *Presentations for Decision Makers*, 4th edn. John Wiley and Sons, New York.

Jay, A. and Jay, R. (1996) *Effective Presentation*. Pitman Publishing, London.

Jeary, T. (1996) *Inspire Any Audience*. Trophy Publishing, Dallas.

Kaplan, B.J. (1997) *A Nurse's Guide to Public Speaking*. Springer Publishing Company, New York.

Kirby, T (1994) *117 Ideas for Better Business Presentations*. The Executive Speaker Company, Dayton, Oh.

Kliem, R.L. and Ludin, I.S. (1995) *Stand and Deliver*. Gower, Aldershot.

Krannich, C.R. (1998) *101 Secrets of Highly Effective Speakers*. Impact Publications, Vermont.

Kroeger, I. (1997) *The Complete Idiot's Guide to Successful Business Presentations*. Alpha Books, New York.

Leary, M. (1993) *Understanding Social Anxiety: Social, Personality and Clinical Perspectives*. Sage Publications, Beverly Hills, Ca.

Leigh, A. and Marnard, M. (1993) *The Perfect Presentation*. Arrow Business Books, London.

Lewis, E. SE. (1936) *Going to Make a Speech?* The Ronal Press Company, New York.

Lowe, D. (1994) *PowerPoint for Windows for Dummies*. IDG Books, San Mateo, Ca.

McCarthy, E.H. (1989) *Speechwriting*. The Executive Speaker Company, Dayton, Oh.

McMillan, I. and Mangan, P. (1998) Effective writing skills for nurses. *Nursing Times*.

Mehrabian, A. (1972) *Non Verbal Communication*. Aldine Atherton, Chicago.

Molloy, J.T. (1996) *New Woman's Dress for Success Book*. Warner Books, New York.

Monkhouse, B. (1988) *Just Say a Few Words – The Complete Speaker's Handbook*. Lennard Publishing, Harpenden.

Pease, A. (1997) *Body Language*, 3rd edn. Sheldon Press, London.

Peoples, D.A. (1992) *Presentations Plus*. John Wiley & Sons, New York.

Peyton, J.W.R. (1998) *Teaching and Learning in Medical Practice*. Manticore Europe Ltd., Rickmansworth.

Pike, B. and Arch, D. (1997) *Dealing with Difficult Participants*. Jossey-Bass/Pfieffer, San Francisco, Ca.

Quilliam, S. (1997) *Body Language Secrets*. Thorsons, London.

Rawlins, K. (1993) *Presentation and Communication Skills*. Macmillan, London.

Ringle, W.J. (1998) *TechEdge – Using Computers to Present and Persuade*. Allyn and Bacon, Needham Heights, Ma.

Robbins, J. (1997) *High Impact Presentations*. John Wiley & Sons, New York.

Sarnoff, D. (1972) *Speech Can Change Your Life*. Doubleday and Co., New York.

Seyle, H. (1975) *Stress Without Distress*. Cygnet Books, New York.

Sheridan, D.R. and Dowdney, D.L. (1997) *How to Write and Publish Articles in Nursing*, 2nd edn. Springer, New York.

Spillane, M. (1991) *The Complete Style Guide*. Piatkus, London.

Spillane, M. (1993a) *Presenting Yourself – A Personal Image Guide for Men*. Piatkus, London.

Spillane, M. (1993b) *Presenting Yourself – A Personal Image Guide for Women*. Piatkus, London.

Stevens, M. (1996) *How to be Better at Giving Presentations*. Kogan Page, London.

Stuart, C. (1996) *How to be an Effective Speaker*. NTC Publishing, Chicago.

Stuttard, M. (1997) *The Power of Public Speaking*. Barrons Educational Series, New York.

Theibert, P.R. (1997) *How to Give a Damn Good Speech*. Career Press, Franklin Lakes, NJ.

Thomas, D.A. and Fryar, M. (1987) *Successful Business Speaking*. National Textbook Company, Chicago, Il.

Urech, E. (1997) *Speaking Globally*. Kogan Page, London.

Van Ments, M. (1990) *Active Talk – The Effective Use of Discussion in Learning*. Kogan Page, London.

Veehoff, D.C. (1985) Standing ovation – a holistic approach to public speaking. *Journal of Nursing Administration*, 15 (10): 34–38.

Walters, L. (1995) *What To Say When You're Dying on the Platform*. McGraw-Hill, New York.

Woodall, M.K. (1997) *Presentations That Get Results – 14 reasons Yours May Not*. Professional Business Communication, Lake Oswego, Or.

Wylie, P. and Grothe, M. (1993) *Dealing With Difficult Colleagues*. Piatkus, London.

Index